OUT OF THE WRECKAGE

* The Pop Stories *

by

Barbara Blanks

aka

StFlossie

for Pop, of course

*
*
*

and for Mary Winklebleck,
the best mom
—and toughest editor—
I'll ever have

*
*
*

with special thanks to
the people of the Rubberstampers List who adopted Pop,
and without whom these stories wouldn't have been written.

A FEW COMMENTS FROM RUBBERSTAMPERS
WHO READ THE ORIGINAL POP STORIES

Flossie, the stories you tell about yourself and Pop are a joy to read. The love you have for him shines out of each letter of every word.
Kaz
***

Barb, I've sure been enjoying these stories. Your style reminds me of the woman who wrote "Fried Green Tomatoes." I truly hope you are saving each and every one as they are priceless.
Suzanne
***

Hi Floss,
My dad apparently has Alzheimer's (I'm still somewhat in denial about it), and your posts help me be less upset—not much less upset—but it helps, and I really appreciate it. So your stories have much more importance to them than you probably know.
Nancy
***

Hi Barb, I can't tell you how much joy your stories have brought to my life. I share them with my own children who have never lived near any of their own grandparents.
Stacie
***

Barb, Thanks for sharing with us. I hope Pop realizes how important you have made him to this group! Your stories made me laugh and cry. They're a wonderful tribute to his life.
Fran
***

Re: Pop's biopsy report
Barb, I'm so terribly sorry. Pop reminds me so much of my daddy, and this hurts.
Anne
***

Re: Pop is failing
I wish I had a Pop in my life. I do because of you. I feel Pop is mine. Thank you for being generous enough to share him.
Sharon
***

IN THE BEGINNING

Disrupt my life to take care of my 81-year-old father-in-law? Oh, please!

Didn't matter that I loved him.

Didn't matter that for twenty-eight years he'd been more father to me than my own dad.

Didn't matter that his whole life changed overnight while mine was merely inconvenienced.

Having Pop three minutes up the road would hamper my activities, take up my time, and make him a dominant presence in my existence. I wasn't happy about it.

Like me, an estimated 44 million people provide some level of unpaid care to another adult, either full- or part-time. And like me, new caregivers may fear their lives will be "ruined" by the demands on their time and emotions. It helps to have someone to talk to—and I was lucky.

I often relieved my stress and frustration by talking to a group of people belonging to a subscription Rubberstampers List on the Internet. Writing about Pop helped me focus on him. It shook out my fear and resentment, and let the love and laughter back in.

What I didn't expect was the group's response. From homemaker to lawyer, from student to doctor, they not only encouraged me, but often commented on how reflective of their own experiences Pop's stories were. The RS members wound up adopting him, and he became their dad, grandfather, husband, or father-in-law, too.

Most how-to-cope books focus on the negative aspects of senior care; horror stories abound. *Out of the Wreckage: The Pop Stories* is a love story. While it talks candidly about life and death, and doesn't shy away from the irritations and difficulties of elder care, it chooses to focus on the positive—the fun side.

At the beginning of Pop's and my fifteen-month journey, if you had told me that enhance, enrich and enliven could be positive synonyms for complicate, dominate and aggravate, I would have snorted in disbelief. I never would have thought a life-changing car wreck could be a blessing, but it was. It gave Pop and me time together that we wouldn't have had otherwise.

Out of the wreckage, I learned my feelings were just my feelings. They were neither good nor bad in and of themselves—it's what I did with them that counted.

Out of the wreckage, I learned attitude, not circumstances, made life a joy or a misery.

Out of the wreckage, I learned when love shouldered the burden and laughter lightened the load, even grief was bearable.

And because of Pop's bladder, I also learned the location of almost every restroom in town.

In *Out of the Wreckage* you will see how an uneducated, ordinary man from a small town in Texas became internationally known. His story is universal.

His name was J. D. Blanks.

About the Author

Barbara Blanks claims her odd and twisted trek along the rubberstamping road has led to writing…in an odd and twisted way. Actually, she's just odd and twisted, but she *has* been published in a variety of venues, and has won/placed/showed in story and poetry contests.

Called StFlossie, Flossie, Flossker, and Floozie by her fellow rubberstampers, Barb is known for her exuberant love of life, her pursuit of a sense of direction, and the liberties she often takes with reality. She is also admired for her stick-to-it-iveness, although of late, she mostly sticks to her unmopped kitchen floor.

OUT OF THE WRECKAGE
* THE POP STORIES *

Friday, May 5:

Car wreck

Oh great. Pop wrecked his car—again.

He called us about three hours after it happened, swearing he was all right. In fact, he'd already called a tow truck, his insurance company, and his brother Mark.

Pop's my father-in-law. I'm married to his only son/child, John. He told us he'd just left his girlfriend's house when he swerved to avoid a dog, and drove his Chevy into a tree. He limped back to Nancy Lee's, who treated his wounds and took him home.

He needed us—well, John—to help him rent a car since he doesn't have any credit cards, and you pretty much need one to do that. He lives near Tyler, out in the country, so he has to have a car.

Pop was still in bed when John, Charlie the Dog, and I got to his place this morning. He tried to sit up, yelled in pain, and grabbed his neck. His airbag-punched eighty-one-year-old body had gone down for the count.

We called the paramedics. They strapped him to a backboard, and loaded him into the ambulance. Mark arrived about then, and we went to the hospital emergency room together. While we waited for x-ray results, John and Mark kept wandering in and out of the exam room, too restless to just sit and wait. I was content to stay with Pop because John foraged coffee for me several times.

At one point, they stayed while I went in search of relief because John forages coffee real well. Good thing men can pee in a bottle because Pop was strapped to that board for four hours.

A doctor finally told us Pop's neck appeared unbroken and let him go. He squawked as he shifted from the backboard to the wheelchair, groaning, "I feel like I've been rode hard and put up wet."

Mark immediately reverted from worried adult to tormenting younger-brother mode. He slapped Pop on the shoulder, and whooped, "Giddyup, little buckaroo!"

9

Pop bellowed, as much from surprise as from the blow. He threatened physical harm to Mark—who just cackled about it all the way out to the parking lot.

Pop awkwardly folded himself into the front seat of the car. John found himself wedged against the steering wheel after pulling the driver's seat forward to let in Mark—who still had to corkscrew his legs around to fit into the backseat. When I eased in next to him, it felt like I was scrunched inside a clown's car, which—considering what wisecrackers those three are—isn't a far off simile.

Mark headed back to Longview after seeing his brother settled into his recliner. John drove to Walmart with the prescription for pain pills, and to buy extra food and litter for Miss Kitty, who was about to be left alone for several days. We had to bring Pop home with us since he certainly wasn't in any condition to take care of himself.

I gotta admit the prospect didn't thrill me. Past experience has proven him to be a lousy patient. He moans and groans and acts like he doesn't feel good—which he doesn't—but gee, quit being such a baby.

Truth to tell, I make a lousy nurse. Since I rarely get sick, I'm not very sympathetic. My bedside manner tends to run toward: "What's your problem? Quit whining. Get over it." But Pop thinks I'm wonderful, and I love him, so I try to curb my Nurse Ratchet tendencies.

While John helped his dad get dressed, I discovered the cat formerly known as "Scat! Shoo!" hadn't been using her litter box—probably because it contained only a dusting of litter. She'd made good use of the guest bed and bedroom carpet though. John and I dragged the nasty mattress and filthy bed linens out the backdoor to take to the trash dump another day.

By late afternoon we had filled the car trunk and jammed more stuff behind the driver's seat—I'm too tired to explain about that right now. Pop reclined his seat to let the headrest support his hurting neck. Charlie, our fifty-pound golden retriever/German shepherd mix, hogged two-thirds of the back seat. I played accordion and squeezed myself into the remaining space for the two-and-a-half-hour drive back to Garland.

Now—I told you all that to tell you that if you e-mail me and don't hear back right away, this is why: I have Pop parked in my living room.

Saturday, May 6:

Pop and our unusual situation

We moved Pop into our bedroom last night because it has fastest access to a bathroom—when he's gotta go, he's gotta go. Somewhere around midnight, he staggered out of bed and hit the wall. The crash sent me flying off the couch—where I was trying to sleep—and racing into the bedroom to see if he was all right. John, sleeping in the guest bunk directly across the hall, stayed totally oblivious.

This morning I saw what looked like blood smeared on the bedroom wall. It wasn't. It was dirty skin Pop had scraped off his arm. Oh dear. We knew he'd quit taking showers after he slipped about three years ago—taking out the curtain rod along with the shower curtain—and had started taking sink baths instead. He didn't stink, so we thought he was cleaning himself fairly well, but apparently not.

Well, the main thing right now is Pop is solid bruise from left shoulder to hip—not to mention the black eye. (It's a wonder the air bag didn't break his glasses.) He can't stand without assistance—and I can't assist him. He's too big and heavy—6'2" and as broad across as his recliner. John can't stay home to help—he's going out of town on business for the first time ever. We're going to need help.

Aside from that, I've been doing laundry—ours and his—for the last ten-and-a-half hours. No exaggeration. I had filled three big trash bags with unwashed clothes and bedding Pop had been throwing into his closets. That's why the car was so packed yesterday.

It's midnight again, and I've just folded up the ironing board. Think I'd better fold up myself, too, and get to bed—well, an unreasonable facsimile anyway.

Sunday, May 7:

Pop is moving to Mayberry Homes

Even though we're pressed for time since John leaves for New York in two days, he didn't want to deal with looking for professional help and tried to procrastinate. I got mad. He reluctantly got out the phone book.

The third place he called—Mayberry Assisted Living Homes—said they had one vacancy. John asked what they provided and how much it cost. Pop's social security and IRA income would cover that amount with some left over. Plus, it's just a mile from us, which makes it awfully convenient. Charlie and I have often walked through the field across the street from it, but I'd never paid attention to that group of houses until about two weeks ago. Almost seems prophetic.

An hour later we met Cortney, the young lady who stays at Mayberry Homes on weekends. We didn't take Pop with us in case the place turned out to be a dump—but it's definitely not. Cortney gave us the tour.

When Pam, the owner, arrived, she made it clear Mayberry is not a nursing home. Certain legal restrictions apply: residents can't be bedridden, or have advanced Alzheimer's, for instance. They have to be able to do some things for themselves.

Based on her interview, she said Pop was probably a candidate for residency. Dianne, the manager, would have the final word after she interviewed him tomorrow morning.

If he's accepted, he'll have professional care—and companionship. We know he's been lonely—and sometimes scared—living by himself. He once told John that the reason he drives around so much going nowhere is he hates being alone at home. It's worse for him when the weather is bad because he can't get out; he just sits and broods.

Several times over the last three or four years, we've talked with him about either moving into assisted living or hiring live-in help. He always claimed he wasn't ready for that, even though we could see his physical strength failing along with his memory.

His housekeeping efforts have been going south, as evidenced by all those dirty clothes, and being unaware of his cat not using the litter box. A crisis—something as simple as the lights going out—panics and confuses him. His reflexes are so slow that I've refused to ride in the car if he's driving—he scares the fool out of me—and that takes a lot of scaring. He shouldn't be driving anymore, but he can't live at home and *not* drive.

We don't think it's a coincidence that Mayberry Homes has an opening for him. The reality is Pop needs long-term help, and in acknowledging this, it's like the weight of the world has fallen off John's shoulders.

Not taking action—or not knowing what action to take—is a heavy burden.

Monday, May 8:

Moving to Mayberry

We took turns crying after yesterday's decision was made. Seems like we're a bunch of crybabies, but it was a relief, too.

Pop hasn't been sleeping well—he hurts too much to get comfortable. And even though our bed is only two feet from the half-bath, last night he peed on the carpet because in struggling to get up, he just couldn't hold it long enough to get to the toilet.

We took him to Mayberry Homes this morning. It's a group of four houses surrounded by well-kept gardens in front, and assorted shade and pine trees out back, giving it a cozy, homey feeling. The bonus view from the front porch is a large spring-fed pond—complete with ducks and at least one heron—sparkling just beyond the parking lot fence.

In House 2, an open portal in the kitchen faces the front door so whoever is on duty can see who is entering or leaving. Immediately to the right of the entry is a living room with two overstuffed couches, a big-screen TV and a stereo sound system. The living room flows into the dining room, which also opens to the kitchen, so it's all very spacious. The residents' rooms line the two long hallways—five rooms on each side of the house; eight women and one married couple are already in residence. In the center (behind the kitchen) are the laundry room, shower/bath, a pantry, and storage rooms; all meals and laundry service are provided.

Dianne, the house administrator, interviewed Pop and approved his application. We spent part of the morning filling out forms, then he was shown to Room 10. It was immediately obvious the twin bed wouldn't do—it's too short and narrow for him. So John and I went to a bed store, bought a double bed; went to another store, and bought a recliner. Afterwards, John went to work, and I drove to Walmart to buy bed linens and other supplies.

We checked on Pop this evening. He looked like he wanted to cry, but he's trying to do what he's "supposed" to. He's "trying not to be a bother."

How sad that in not wanting to hurt a dog, his whole life has turned upside down.

It's midnight again.

Tuesday, May 9:

Pop reclines

Pop is still in pain. Dianne, the manager, said several of the ladies went to a Dr. A, so on that recommendation, I called his office. They worked us in today. We had to wait awhile, but Dr. A was worth it—he's cute. Young and yummy and yumpin' yiminy cute!

Oh, umm-m, it's whiplash. Dr. A wrote out a prescription for pain medicine; not much else he could do.

We got back to Mayberry just in time to sign for the new bed. After the delivery men set it up, I ran home to get the linens. Since my big strong man left for New York earlier today, I called Greg-next-door and asked if he could help me get Pop's new chair so he wouldn't have to wait another three days for delivery.

Greg's strong, too—and I was lucky enough to snag another big strong male employee at the store—so I didn't have to do any chair carrying or lifting onto the bed of the pickup. After we got to Mayberry, I must have looked pathetic trying to help Greg, because a big strong gardener grabbed my end—of the chair, that is—and he and Greg carried it inside.

It dwarfs the room. It didn't look that big in the store. There's no handle to operate the footrest either. Pop's having trouble pushing on the arms to get it into recline position. Still, it's more comfortable than sitting on his bed—and he looks quite regal when enthroned.

He said everyone's being real nice to him. Certainly he's enjoying the three meals a day, plus snacks. I took over our old black-and-white TV last night—a stopgap until we can get him color. No remote control either—how primitive. He's decided whatever channel it's on is the channel it stays on—that's easier than getting up to change it. He frequently watches with his eyes closed anyway.

I went home for awhile, called his girlfriend Nancy Lee to give her a status report, then went back to Mayberry after supper with Charlie. He loved exploring the grounds behind the houses. After he wore himself out, we joined Pop on the porch, where he was enjoying the breeze and the view of the pond, as were two of the ladies. I think Miss Bess already likes him.

OK, I want you to know that Pop doesn't lose his sense of humor during dark times—and these are dark times for him. He's joked around a little the last couple of days, but the most dramatic example I can give you is this old story I'm going to tell on him now:

14

Several years ago my mother-in-law Pat had her right leg amputated due to diabetes-caused gangrene. After her surgery, John had to go back to work in Garland, but I stayed on in Tyler to help out, mostly by spelling Pop at the hospital—he was no better at sitting still back then than John and Mark are now.

One evening we had supper together in the hospital cafeteria. Pop usually doesn't say much, but that night he started talking about how much he loved Pat, how "down in the dumps" he'd been, and how much better he felt since I was there. He talked about being a farmer, and how Pat had plowed fields right beside him; how when she got pregnant with John, he took a job making $1.05/day so he could support them better; and he told me how Pat had taken care of his mother when she was dying of cancer.

During his monologue, he was working on a huge taco salad. He had eaten about half when he got this wry grin on his face.

"You know, Barbara," he said in his gruff voice, "I think they get this ground meat from amputated limbs."

"Pop!" I cried, pretending shock. "You could be eating Mother's leg!"

"No-o-o-o," he mused. "I think she was in Monday's soup."

We laughed over that. Sometimes you have to laugh so you don't cry. And we've had our moments of laughter even during these last difficult days.

Sunday, May 14:

Pop settles in

John got home from New York Thursday evening. On Friday we drove to Tyler with a long list of errands to do for Pop. We didn't take him because we could just flat move faster without him.

We set up mail forwarding, and subscribed to mail delivery of the Tyler newspaper. When we went to clean out the car, the wrecker told us Pop hit the tree so hard he'd actually broken the engine. I haven't seen the tree, but I bet it'll never be the same either.

From there we stopped at the insurance company to finalize Pop's claim. Finally, we went to Lowe's and Walmart for padlocks for the storage sheds, security-light timers, more cat litter, and other stuff. Back at the house we consoled Charlie for having left him alone with Miss Kitty. Felines make him nervous—actually, he's afraid of them, but that's another story.

John got to work cutting the grass. Although I'd surfaced-cleaned for Pop last November, it didn't involve opening drawers, cupboards or closets. This time it did. I pulled out massive quantities of assorted papers, worn-out clothes and linens, out-dated foods in cupboards and the fridge—not that there was much food on hand besides boxes of Little Debbie brownies. I filled seven plastic bags with trash, and four brown-paper grocery sacks with papers to sort through later.

John continued working outside on Saturday, but I spent most of that day with my mom—she lives in Tyler, too. We ran a couple of errands, ran into a couple of yard sales, and ran our mouths.

Late Saturday afternoon John and I packed the car to the gills, squeezed in the dog—sorry, Charlie—and cast off for home.

Today, while doing the last loads of Pop's laundry, I threw away clothes that were too stained to come clean, or too torn or worn out to mend. During the last ten years of living alone, he developed his own style of washing and mending: throw it in the closet and close the door.

Ya know, I'm beginning to think he had the right idea.

Friday, May 19:

Thursday in the park with Pop

He must be feeling better. He's a little restless, a little bored, and a little tired of remote-less black-and-white TV. He didn't exactly complain about it when I saw him after work on Monday, but close.

On Tuesday I set up a local checking account for him and took paperwork for him to sign. I'd have taken him to the bank with me, but I was meeting friend Anne for our monthly lunch/visit/shop date and needed to move fast.

On Wednesday John bought a color TV—with remote! We set it atop Pop's dresser because that gave him the best view from a reclining position. Unfortunately the stations aren't coming in too clearly—it needs an antenna-connecting cable. At least he can flip through the static while he reads his Tyler paper—the first one arrived in the mail.

Thursday morning Charlie and I went to Mayberry, intent on making it up to Pop for neglecting him on Tuesday. We found him in bed, fully clothed. He'd eaten breakfast, then crawled back under the covers. He said he was resting. I think he's depressed. Told him we had some fun in store, prodded him out of bed, and drove a couple of miles to a city park with a pond.

We had to park on the street. Crossing a wide, grassy downslope between the curb and sidewalk was the only way to get to the deck overlooking the pond. Negotiating that with a walker—oh, I guess I should mention Pop has been using Mother Pat's old walker since his accident. Anyway, maneuvering down the slope wasn't easy with a frenzied, still-on-leash dog underfoot. However, aside from Charlie getting stepped on a couple of times, we made it without casualties.

I unleashed Crazy Dog, who proceeded to chase squirrels, tried to climb the trees after them, then raced around the pond trying to retrieve the ducks without actually jumping into the water. Pop had as much fun watching Charlie as Charlie had exhausting himself. After all that excitement, we still got back to Mayberry in time for lunch.

OK, two things: Pop has been more a father to me these last twenty-eight years than my own dad, whom I haven't seen in as many years. (My dad's in Detroit, and while we write regularly, we're not close.) He and Mother Pat welcomed me with open arms when I married their son—the fact that he loved me was good enough for them. Her arms stayed around me until she died. Pop's are still there.

He's more needy than usual right now, and quite honestly, sometimes it's difficult to deal with—for John especially. Pop usually won't come right out and say what he wants, then is hurt when he doesn't get it. He tells us we don't need to come see him every day, then thinks we're mad at him if we don't, which is frustrating and aggravating. He needs something to do, but he's not interested in trying anything we've suggested. He's never had to develop his own inner resources, so without work, driving or puttering around his property, he's completely dependent on others for entertainment.

These last several days Pop's been playing "poor pitiful me" with John—and John resents it. He's spent time with his dad almost every day since the accident, mostly after a long day at work. In addition, he has the wife and dog—who usually see Pop during the day—waiting at home, and feeling neglected in the evening. John needs time for himself, too, but he's getting almost none.

We *are* going to find a balance here. We're learning a new way of life, and it's rough at times, but it'll be OK.

The second thing is: while going through some of the papers I brought back from Pop's house last weekend, I came across his old Army Air Force identification badge from 1942. It shows a handsome, slender man, full head of wavy hair, shoulders thrown back, clear-eyed and alert. It's easy to see why the first time Mother Pat saw him she said, "That's the man I'm going to marry."

Now he's bent and stooped, gray where he's not bald, broadened, and wrinkled. It seems impossible that he's the same person as in that picture, but next time I visit him, I'm going to try real hard to see that young man.

Pop's given name, by the way, is John. He reminds me of a Robert Burns poem:

> John Anderson my jo, John,
> When first we were acquent,
> Your locks were like the raven
> Your bonie brow was brent;
> But now your brow is beld, John,
> Your locks are like the snaw;
> But blessings on your frosty pow,
> John Anderson, my jo!

brent is smooth, unwrinkled
pow is head
jo is Scottish for sweetheart

And Pop is a sweetheart, in spite of his occasional cranky ways —which he inherited from his son. I'm never cranky. Ha.

Friday, May 26:

Pop-a-doodle-doo!

Last Saturday John went to Tyler to cut the grass, among other chores. He didn't get home till late, so I visited with his dad after supper. Talked with some of the ladies, too—they've been feeding his ego by telling him how sweet he is.

"I'm the only rooster in the hen house," was his smug way of explaining his popularity, which he certainly enjoys. Well, the only single rooster. One married man lives there with his wife of sixty-some years.

It's been a long week—seems that way at least. Even though John and I have been to Mayberry several times, or been there to bring him here, Pop's having a rough time.

Tuesday morning I picked up a prescription and took it to Pop. That night I talked John out of going over after work, urging him to cut himself some slack. I went instead and wound up staying two hours. Dianne told me Pop hadn't gotten dressed all day, nor did he eat lunch. No appetite? He's definitely depressed.

"Would a phone in your room make you feel better?" I asked. "You wouldn't have to use the house phone and could call us—or Nancy Lee and Mark—any time you wanted." That definitely sounded good to him.

Today I arranged to have the phone line in his room turned on. John took our spare phone over later—it'll do until we can bring his cordless up from Tyler. Pop is once again connected to the world.

Wednesday, May 31:
Pop cracked open his head this morning

He'd been flipping his walker upward as he sauntered through the kitchen to get to the breakfast table—showing off for the ladies is what he was doing. He lost his balance and toppled backward.

I was about to leave our house when Dianne called, so I detoured to Mayberry. As I rushed in, I noticed the other ten residents sitting around the tables, not eating their breakfasts and not speaking. They were just watching Pop, who was sitting on a chair someone had moved into the kitchen. All eyes turned toward me.

"Good morning," I said brightly. No one responded. It was eerie, but I didn't hear any spooky music, so I kept moving forward.

Aside from being embarrassed, Pop said he felt OK, but the skin was split open at the crown of his head, and wouldn't stop bleeding. He's hard-headed, but the kitchen floor was harder. Not knowing what else to do, I took him to the emergency room.

He dabbed at the blood with a tissue during the drive to the hospital. He said his head didn't hurt, but when the doctor gave him a shot to numb his scalp, he winced and yelped. I started laughing; he gave me a sheepish grin.

The doctor said I did the right thing bringing Pop in because scalp wounds have a tendency to keep opening up if not stitched—and it took eight to close the wound.

"Hey, Pop, we're going to get you in the next Frankenstein movie," I said. "You can be the monster!"

"OK," he grumbled, "but can I get something to eat first?"

That's right! The poor man never got his breakfast.

Back at Mayberry, I scrounged some food for him, then left to run those errands I'd intended running three hours earlier. Stopped by to check on him afterwards. He was doing fine—no hallucinations, no more bleeding, but there's a big ol' goose egg on the top of his head. He kept reaching up to feel his stitches. If he's not careful, he's liable to untie himself.

Got home just as Mona, my occasional boss, was leaving a message asking if I could work the next two days. I grabbed the receiver and told her I could, but I'd have to come in late since Pop had doctor's appointments both mornings.

To top off the day, Charlie developed a bloody diarrhea—probably a reaction to an anti-inflammatory he's been taking for his hurt knee. (He twisted it a few days ago when another dog tried to attack him while we were on our walk.) John and I rushed him to the vet's office just before it closed. The poor baby got two shots, but he didn't wince *or* yelp—unlike some people I could mention.

Oh yeah, John's been wanting us to get a cell phone. My attitude has been, "No, No, No! We don't *need* a cell phone." But circumstances have changed. If Dianne hadn't caught me this morning, she would have called John, who would have had to leave work. So we're getting a cell phone.

And just so you know, when John went to Tyler Sunday, he brought back Pop's—actually Mother Pat's—old blue recliner to replace that new one we'd bought. It was just too big for his room. Pop's old chair feels like home and fits him just fine.

Friday, June 2:

Never a dull moment

And now for the continuing saga of Pop, soon to be a soap opera near you...

The day before he fell I'd spent all morning on the phone setting up appointments with new doctors, and contacting his old doctors to have his records transferred here. He was already past due for his glaucoma check-up, plus he had commented that he was having some trouble reading, so his vision needed testing, too. We went to see his new ophthalmologist yesterday morning.

Several people at Mayberry liked Dr. H, and I suppose he was good—certainly he was better than the bozo I went to three years ago who was so overbooked that it took him five hours to examine me. He'd do one test, race off to another patient or two, return to me to do another test, disappear, come back—you get the idea.

Dr. H had assistants who did all the basic grunt work before he came into the exam room for about two minutes and did some glaucoma measurement. Someone put drops in Pop's eyes before leading us to a darkened room to watch a video about glaucoma and cataracts while we waited for his pupils to dilate.

What we got was fifteen minutes of *loud* commercials for Disney products. Excuse me, but I don't want to sit through *loud* commercials at a doctor's office—or any commercials for that matter. It really annoyed me. Eventually a very short *loud* video about glaucoma came on. Pop wasn't bothered because he can't hear too well anyway, but I had my fingers in my ears the entire time. I wonder if Dr. H is associated with a hearing-loss clinic.

We were finally led to another room. The doc came in again for about three minutes to finish the exam and give his proclamation. Pop's glaucoma is under control, but he's developing cataracts.

We were there for two-and-a-half hours, most of it waiting, which is not my strong suit. I have a problem with doctors who are too busy for their patients. My middle name is "Let's move it!" Pop's easier going than I am.

Also, his pace isn't fast, but he does the best he can. We both noticed the poorly concealed impatience displayed by some of the assistants over his slow walk, which ticked me off. He tried to hurry, but even his hurry is slow. Young never thinks it's going to get old.

After taking him back to Mayberry, I dashed home to let Charlie out to do his business, then grabbed a sandwich before heading off to work.

Today Pop had an appointment with Dr. A, his new family doctor. We were there for two-and-a-half hours, too, but I enjoyed The View this time. Also, I was smart enough to take *RubberStamp-*

Madness, a stamping magazine, with me. While we were waiting for Hunka-Doctor to come into the exam room, I passed it to Pop. He looked through it carefully, not really understanding what it was about, but I told him that was the kind of thing I liked to do, and that was good enough for him.

Doctor A-mazingly Cute never seemed to rush through any part of the exam. He looked at me when he needed some details filled in, but he talked directly to Pop most of the time, which I'm discovering is not the norm. Too often people assume because he's old, he's stupid or senile. He's neither.

Dr. A did a complete skin check after finding a misshapen black mole on Pop's chest, which he shaved off for biopsy. He also wanted x-rays taken before prescribing physical therapy for Pop's neck—especially since he'd recently crash-landed in Mayberry's kitchen.

So we toddled over to Radiology. The x-ray tech was wonderfully patient, even when she needed to re-do two shots because Pop couldn't hold his head up high enough for her to get good pictures.

"Is there anything I can do to help?" I asked. Famous last words.

She slipped a long, lead-lined "dress" over me—must have weighed three hundred pounds. OK, so maybe only two hundred-fifty.

She had me stand behind Pop and hold up his left arm (it has tendon-damage, and he can't raise it very high by himself.) She told him to lower his right shoulder. For some reason, trying to relax his shoulder made him relax his knees. He started sinking down and backward, which made him panic. He yelled, "Don't let me fall! Don't let me fall!"

"Straighten your legs, Pop!" I was pressed against his back trying to support him, but he was too heavy, and with the added weight of the "dress," I was sinking down with him.

"Straighten your legs!" I shouted again, loudly enough to get through to him. He straightened his legs and regained his balance... pant pant puff puff. Man! I don't know about him, but I was sweating.

Got one x-ray taken.

The tech needed him to raise his chin, but he couldn't maintain that position because it made his neck hurt. She had me press my hand against his forehead to hold the tilt, but even then he couldn't raise it much.

Once again I dropped Pop off at Mayberry—well, I went in search of food first since he'd missed lunch. Turned out Gabriella, the daytime house "mother," saved a plate for him, bless her. Repeat the scene at home: Charlie out, grab a sandwich, head for work.

While I was gone, the doctor's office left a message saying the x-rays were still unclear, so Pop's scheduled for a CT scan next Thursday. Stay tuned…

Thursday, June 8:
How to tell when you're really tired

Prologue: Miss Bess bought a cinnamon-red Olds Cutlass Ciera when she was 82. She put only 21,000 miles on it before moving into Mayberry when she was 91. It's been parked in her daughter Brenda's garage for the last month and was up for sale.

Our truck has over 100,000 miles on it, and my flaming-red Dodge has almost 80,000. So we took the Olds for a test drive. It's larger than the Dodge, and Pop should be able to get into it more easily. Plus, it has cool automatic just-about-everything. No more cranking window handles!

It seemed in super condition, but we wanted it checked over anyway. When we picked it up, we tried to leave Pop with Brenda as a security deposit, but she wanted a check. Hmph.

Our mechanic suggested a radiator flush, transmission service, and replacement of some belts and hoses that were dried out. He said the original tires had plenty of tread, but were cracked from age; we'd need to get new ones. Still, the car was a deal.

Today's agenda:

—Call Brenda and agree on final price of the car, then call shop and OK the work they suggested.

—Go to shop to get stuff out of trunk and glove compartment to return to Brenda. Car is up on rack having transmission fluid drained. Have mechanic lower rack. Get old floor mats out of trunk and don't notice bottom of one is oily. Get oil on your shirt, but forget to change it every time you go home.

—Go to Brenda's house to deliver stuff, pay for car and get title.

—Drive across town to insurance company to get title transfer form, because you were smart enough to call to see if they had one in order to avoid going to county tax office for it. Also give agent enough info to get insurance process started.

—Drive half-way back across town to have owner (Miss Bess) sign title and transfer form.

—Drive back across town to tax office. As you stand in line, read the sign over the Information Desk listing items needed to transfer title, realize you failed to write down license tag number of new car, can't remember the shop's phone number so you can call to ask them, and drive all the way home to get number off business card—because you didn't think to look in a phone book at the tax office. Nor did you think to look at the bumper sticker on the Dodge which also has their number.

—Have that pointed out to you by the snickering manager of the shop before he tells you the new license plate number.

—Drive to the grocery store because you haven't bought groceries in two weeks and the cupboards are bare. Drive home, put up groceries, then have mechanic call to say the Olds is ready.

—Call best friend Nan, who lives practically across the street from you, ask her to take you to get car, because even though you've walked that mile to the shop before, right now a mile is too far in the afternoon heat.

—Drive back to insurance company in new car to finish getting new insurance coverage, and be glad you were accidentally smart enough to do that since the tax office will ask for proof of insurance, an item you didn't notice on their check list when you were there earlier.

—Drive to tax office again. Be grateful it's not crowded, and be especially grateful that the set-up has changed, which means once the Information Desk goes through your papers, they give you a number and you can sit down until it's your turn, but is that nearly as much fun as the former stand-in-line-until-the-blood-leaves-your-head-and-you-pass-out method? Well, yes! Of *course* it is!

—Try to read the book you brought since you expected to wait a long time, but get bounced around on the bench seat by two kids at the other end who are unable to sit still.

—Get title transferred at last. Proud new owner of new car deserves reward.

—Drive across town again—but west this time instead of north and south—because you are desperate for a haircut. Park in front of hair salon and try to open car door. It's locked.

—You have automatic door locks now—cool! Hit the Lock button and try to open door again. It's still locked.

—Hit the Lock button again and try to open door. It's still locked. Repeat scene once more.

—Sit there and think, "Oh great. The electrical system has failed. It's a broiling hot day. I am going to roast in my new car. Barbecued Barb in an Olds. Fricasseed Flossie in a Ciera."

—Hit Lock button again. Door still won't open.

—See the light dawn.

—Hit the UNlock button. Door opens.

When the brain quits working, go home and lie down. But get your hair cut first.

Friday, June 9:

A month, a mole and Mayberry

This morning I had tires put on our "new" car—a car we wouldn't have known about except for John and me being friendly with the other Mayberry residents, which is unusual according to Dianne. Most relatives and friends interact only with their resident. That's sad, because not only do those ladies have stories to tell, but they're funny and still full of life.

After the new wheels were on, I test drove Pop to the optical center to have his glasses adjusted, then took him for a haircut. He was getting so shaggy people thought I was hanging out with a hippie.

Later, when Dr. A's nurse called to say that biopsied mole was cancerous, I went back to Mayberry to let Pop know. We walked to the end of the parking lot and back, just to enjoy the glorious afternoon filled with cool sunshine;

You know, it's been just over a month since Pop's accident. When we first moved him up here, I was relieved that we so quickly and easily found good assisted living nearby—partly for his sake, partly for ours. Now I'm reaping an unexpected bonus.

Pop and I have rarely had one-on-one time in the twenty-eight years I've been married to his son. Without the stress of taking care of him full time, I'm really enjoying him when we're together. Not only does he have a delightful sense of humor, but his intelligence and awareness of current events compensate for his lack of formal education. (He dropped out of school in the eighth grade to help his mother with their farm after his father died.)

I've loved Pop for a long time. Now I know I like him, too.

Wednesday, June 14:

Pop hears a Woo-o-o!

His left hearing aid broke a couple of weeks ago. I'd taken it in for repair, and it was finally ready. He wanted me to go to Miracle Ear without him and carry it back, but I told him he could stick it in his ear and carry it himself.

"Is that any way to talk to an old man?" he said, amusement in his voice. But he was ready to go by the time I got to Mayberry. He likes getting out even when he won't admit it.

George the Technician put a new battery in the repaired hearing aid, then checked the other one. No wonder Pop couldn't hear—not only was it crammed full of earwax, but the battery was dead.

He'd forgotten how to clean them, and I never knew, so George gave us a lesson. He also taught us how to balance the volume. It's easy: rub the palms of the hands together near one ear, then the other. Based on the sound levels, turn the knobs toward the nose to raise the volume, and toward the back of the head to lower it.

With both hearing aids working properly, Pop, for the first time in several years, could hear me when I spoke in my normal voice. Woo-o-o! It almost made me cry, it was that wonderful. He could even hear me over the road noise as we drove back to Mayberry.

He decided to sit out in the living room for awhile. Before leaving, I asked if he remembered how to test the volume balance. After a little memory jogging, he rubbed his palms together near each ear.

"This one is a little low," he said. "Should I turn it up?"

"Yes," I prompted, "turn it towards your nose."

He lifted his hand and touched his nose as if to remind himself where it was. I laughed.

"Yep, Pop, your nose is still in the same place it's always been."

He looked a little startled, like he hadn't realized what he was doing, then he laughed, too. He adjusted the volume, tested it again, and was satisfied. I gave him a hug as I got ready to leave, and couldn't resist teasing him.

"Hey, Pop, where's your nose?"

He touched his ear!

Thursday, June 15:

Pop's CT scan adventure

Early this morning I drove Pop to what *used* to be the front entrance of the Garland hospital, which turned out to be the wrong entrance, but we didn't know that until after I walked him inside and saw it was the Discharge area. Sat him down in a chair by the window, told him "I'll be back" in my best Arnold Schwarzenneger voice, trying to inspire confidence in both of us, and left to park the car.

I got lost. When I came back in through a side entrance, I couldn't find my way to Discharge; had to reverse direction, exit the building, and walk around to whateverthehell-side-except-thefrontside of the building it was now.

Pop's face brightened considerably when he saw me finally reappear. Knowing my proclivity for getting lost, he said, "I've been sitting here wondering what I'd do if you didn't come back for me." Bless his heart.

By then we were almost late for his appointment—like they'd process him on time anyway, but I have this thing about not being late. Since it was a long-ish walk to Out-Patient Admitting, I asked for a wheelchair at the Discharge window—which really *did* make us late because we had to wait for the Candy Striper to bring it. I made Pop push me because I was worn out by then. No, no, I pushed him—doing wheelies all the way.

Of course, we still had to wait. Out-Patient got him processed, and gave us the paperwork. We followed a volunteer guide to Special Imaging. Its tiny waiting room was full, and I ran over a few toes before finding a place to park Pop. Still, we didn't have to wait too long before they called him back and ran him through the CT tube, which didn't take long either. They wouldn't let me go with him, but they returned him no worse for wear.

After detouring him to a restroom, we—notice I say "we"—managed to find our way back to the door that actually opened onto the right parking lot. While I brought the car around, he sat outside and soaked up the Texas-heat after the hospital-cold.

Then again, he might have wanted to be a landmark for me.

Friday, June 23:

Pop's cat and other company

We've been trying to find a new home for Miss Kitty. She's still in Tyler, by herself most of the time. Mayberry would allow Pop to keep her in his room, but he's too slow and forgetful—she'd get loose in no time. We can't chance having her scratch or bite someone, or having a resident trip over her.

We can't keep her ourselves. She associates me with the dog that periodically invades her Tyler home and wants nothing to do with me—or the dog. In addition, Charlie's scared of cats. He tried to play with some kittens when he was a puppy, got scratched, and has never recovered from the "abuse." He also has epilepsy, and stress can throw him into a seizure.

We've been in contact with several "rescue" places, and "Texas Cares" called last Saturday. They have an opening at one of their placement centers, but Miss Kitty would have to get her shots and be spayed before they'd accept her. Pop never took care of any of that.

John will bring her to Garland after he returns from New York—again. His company wants him there for three days for more training. The night before he left, we took Pop out for supper. He wanted to cruise around afterwards, so I had them drop me off at home first. Partly I thought it'd be nice if they had some private time together—sounds generous of me, doesn't it? Truth is I just didn't want to drive around aimlessly for an undetermined length of time.

John left for New York Monday morning; I picked up Pop for his new urologist's appointment. His chief complaint is having to get up several times during the night to use the bathroom. Dr. S asked him a lot of questions, drew blood for a PSA test, but didn't actually physically examine him, preferring to wait until he got records from Pop's old doctor.

Yesterday we saw that cutie-patootie Dr. A. Yeah, I took a closer inventory of the man doctor. For some reason he mentioned his age.

"How old did you say you are?" I asked.

"32," he said.

"Oh God," I wailed, "I'm old enough to be your mother!"

Darn! So much for fun fantasies. That aside, the CT scan showed several arthritis spurs, some of which were beginning to compress Pop's spinal cord, but it wasn't clear enough to show what Dr. A really wanted to see. He decided to send them to an expert—a specialist who will have the final say about prescribing physical therapy.

He did decide it wasn't necessary to excise the flesh around the cancerous mole right now. We just need to keep an eye on the area.

John was supposed to get home Wednesday night, but his flight from NY was cancelled because of thunderstorms. Trust me, he wasn't thrilled about having to "sleep" on the airport floor. And he missed the family reunion fun at Mayberry.

Mark and his son had driven up from Longview for a visit. Pop called to ask if I could come over. He and Mark were heavy into cutting up with each other, as brothers will do. Pop was grinning so hard I thought his teeth were going to pop out.

Longview's a three-hour drive from Garland. Mark and Mark, Jr. stayed maybe one-and-a-half hours, then left just as the sky started falling, and continued falling most of the night.

Pop, however, was floating way above Cloud 9, and all was sunshine and rainbows up there.

Thursday, June 29:

Pop's got wheels!

Dr. J is a physiatric (not "psychiatric") doctor, meaning she determines what kind and how much physical therapy a patient needs. She's quiet spoken, with a gentle manner, and has soft crinkles around her eyes from smiling. She asked Pop a lot of questions—about his emotional state as well as his physical.

Because his head tilts to the left, she's concerned that he might have a slipped vertebra that's not showing up on the CT scan. She wants him to have an MRI before she'll prescribe physical therapy.

She watched him walk down the hall and back, then lengthened his walker legs as much as possible—we didn't realize they could be adjusted. He can stand upright almost enough to see where he's going.

She also let him try a walker with wheels on the front legs. He liked it so well that we stopped at a nearby medical supplies pharmacy and ordered a pair. They came in this morning. I went to Mayberry and found him sitting on the front porch.

"Hey, Pop, I'm taking your walker—want to go with it?"

"Well, sure!"

I like a man who's ready to go on a moment's notice—and after he finished going, we drove to the pharmacy.

The pharmacist attached the wheels for us, and we rolled back to the car. We took care of a couple of other errands before we went back to Mayberry. As Pop started walking towards the front door, he ran one wheel off the edge of the concrete.

"When you learn to drive that thing," I said, "I'll get you a horn —unless you'd rather tinkle a bicycle bell."

"I tinkle enough as it is, thank you," he groused.

OK, I wasn't going to tell y'all this, but I need to. Pop acted real chipper when I picked him up, but we were no sooner out of the parking lot than he started crying. I couldn't understand a lot of what he was saying, but the gist of it was he was sorry he was such a burden to John and me, and he just wanted to go to sleep and never wake up again.

Oh, man—tore my heart out. Pop worked hard all his life to take care of his family—as farmer, soldier, roughneck in the oil fields, machinist—and now he can barely take care of himself.

He said he knows there's no going back, and he has to live his life as it is now. Still, not only has he lost the hope that he could ever live at home again, but he has to accept the impending loss of his fur baby.

John brought Miss Kitty up from Tyler last Tuesday so we could start prepping her for "Texas Cares" placement. We took her over to see Pop first. She was nothing but scared, but he thought she'd forgotten him because she spent most of her time trying to hide under his bed. He said that made him feel a little better about giving her up, but he smiled so hard when he *was* able to hold her that it was all I could do to not cry.

After he said his good-byes, John and I took her directly to our vet's.

I feel like such a rat.

Saturday, July 8:

Pop's MRI

John dropped us off at the underground entrance to Baylor Dallas this afternoon, and went to park the car. Pop and I decided that waiting for him just inside the outside door in the alcove was the better part of going through the inner door, on the other side of which were the elevators. Baylor Dallas is an awfully big place to get lost in, even if you're just going Up.

After John joined us, we found our way to the right department. I filled out the paperwork since I now have all Pop's information memorized. We were led to the MRI waiting room, where he was stuck inside a tiny changing closet, made smaller by John going inside to help him disrobe, then en-robing him in hospital gown and paper slippers. Good thing Pop's not closet-ophobic.

One person was allowed to go in the MRI room with him. I had less metal on me than John—just my wedding ring—so it was easier for me to slip that off, and don a gown over my clothes. The MRI tube was huge overall, but the inner tube where Pop was lying was drinking-straw narrow. Good thing he's not suck-ophobic. Or claustrophobic.

The techs sat me as far away from the tube as the room allowed, then went into their protected control room. I had no idea MRIs were so loud or I'd have stripped John of his metal and let him have all the fun. I had to cover my ears each time a picture-taking session started. John claims I have dog ears, so loud noises really do bother me.

Every time the racket stopped, I walked over to pat Pop's ankle —that's about all I could see of him—and offered encouragement. Actually, I think he might have dozed off, because the first time I patted him, he jerked. He probably would have hit his head if they hadn't strapped it down. He told me afterwards that he could feel someone touching him, but couldn't hear anyone talking.

As we were leaving, John got turned around and had to—Gasp!—ask someone for directions. I know it's tacky of me to gloat, but I love it when that happens to him for a change.

Anyway, we filled up at a cafeteria before taking Pop back to Mayberry. He's not the least bit food-ophobic.

Tuesday, July 11:

Pop's cat and other news

Poor Miss Kitty looked pathetic after her physical, shots and spaying. I tried to finger-stroke her through the cat-carrier slots while driving her to the "Texas Cares" adoption location, but she wanted nothing to do with me.

She was placed in one of ten cages set inside a glassed-in room, which keeps customers from casually harassing the cats—only TC volunteers have the door key. Being semi-isolated from all the noise and activities of the store probably makes it a little easier on the cats, too.

But Kitty lasted only four days. As best we understood it, a volunteer had her out of her cage, on a table, trying to brush some of the flea-foam out of her fur, when something startled her. As she leaped off the table, the volunteer grabbed her hind leg, and when Kitty reached the end of her downward arc, she used the woman's leg as a scratching post.

It really wasn't Miss Kitty's fault, but they decided she wasn't a good candidate for a normal adoption after all. Now what? We couldn't keep her—I was adamant about that. Sorry. Not even for Pop. This is Charlie's home, and I won't have him stressed out.

We can't leave her in Tyler, and we can't/won't just turn her loose. No one we've asked locally wants her. John thought the only option left was to have her put down and dreaded telling his dad. That's when I thought of boarding her at our vet's, at least for awhile—to give us a little time to regroup.

So that's where she is now. I went to see her yesterday, taking Charlie with me, partly because he likes everyone there, partly hoping he'd react differently. Nope. He did his Ray Charles impression—shaking his head from side to side ("No, No, No!")—as he tried to back away from her. So much for that.

Meanwhile, Pop's been busy. Dianne said he's socializing quite a bit. He likes all that female attention. John brought him here on the 4th of July, where he sat on the patio and ate my homemade peanut butter cookies.

We also went back to the ophthalmologist's one day. Since I was ranting about it last time, I forgot to tell you Dr. H thought Pop's glaucoma was being over-medicated. He took him off one eye drop and reduced the potency of a second. This exam was to make sure his eye pressure hadn't gone up again. It hadn't.

Sunday, July 16:
Fun with Mom—and Pop, too

My mom was scheduled for cataract surgery on the twelfth. She didn't think I needed to be with her since it's routine nowadays, but I wouldn't listen to her. I haven't for years—why start now?

John thinks I'm directionally impaired just because I get lost a lot. Even though it's a fairly straightforward drive, he didn't entirely trust me to find my way to Tyler, so he decided to take vacation time and go with me—which, of course, meant Pop wanted to go, too. We caravaned down there Tuesday afternoon—the men in the truck, Charlie and me in the car. We needed both vehicles because I planned to stay with Mom at her apartment while John and Pop batched it at his place.

The advances that have been made in cataract surgery are eye-popping. Ha-ha. It took about ninety minutes to process Mom—paperwork, measuring the left eye curvature, eye drops, more eye drops, and more eye drops (mostly numbing the eye, I think). Then they sedated her and fifteen minutes later she was in recovery.

The nurse handed me a fanny pack filled with instructions, a bottle of moisturizing eye drops, a prescription for antibiotic eye drops, a plastic eye shield to use whenever Mom slept for the next seven days, and a pair of extra-dark wraparound sunglasses.

Just as well I was there because instructions were given while the patient was still loopy. She remembered squat later—which was kind of cool, because I could tell her anything. "Yes, Mom, you have to stick your finger in your ear so the eye drops won't leak out that way." She almost believed me.

33

As it turned out, she couldn't manage to get the drops in her eye, so I had to dose her—and she thought she wouldn't need me. Ha. We returned to the clinic the next afternoon for a follow-up exam. All looked well. She's due for another check-up in two weeks, at which time they'll schedule surgery on her right eye.

Mom is good company. When we weren't at the eye clinic, we talked, ran errands, played games, and hit some yard sales on Friday and Saturday mornings. But summer in Texas is miserably hot (near or over 100) and humid (think sauna), so we never stayed out long.

She's still real sharp at 77 because she's always kept her mind active, but she poops out easily. I expected her to sleep a lot which would allow me to work on the embroidery piece I had with me, and to read my backlogged stamping magazines. But she took only one nap each day, and then it was so quiet in her apartment that I wound up nodding off shortly after I picked up the embroidery or opened a magazine.

As for Pop, he visited with Nancy Lee, saw Mark, puttered around his house, and spent lots of time with John. Thursday night Mom and I joined them for supper, after which we intended to play dominoes, but we no sooner settled into a game than company arrived.

Charla is, I think, Pop's second cousin—the daughter of a first cousin anyway. She, her husband Michael, and their two little boys saw our vehicles as they drove by and stopped to say Hi.

I hadn't seen the boys since they were toddlers. Now Josh was six or seven, talkative, aggressive and not at all shy. Jake was about five, very solemn, quiet and sensitive. When they got a little wild (bored with adult conversation), Pop reached into his wallet and gave each a five dollar bill.

Jake wandered over to me, proudly holding the bill in front of him.

"Want to see a disappearing trick?" I asked him. Nod nod nod.

"Give me that," I said, taking the bill. I folded it up while saying, "Abracadabra, Presto, Gone-o!" and very obviously put it into my back pocket. I showed Jake my empty hands.

"See? All gone." Jake stood there, not knowing what to say or do. Josh wandered over just then. "Want to see a disappearing trick?" I asked him. Nod nod nod. (All the adults started paying attention.)

Same deal: "Abracadabra, Presto, Gone-o!" I folded the bill, and put it in my other back pocket. Josh is hip.

"You put it in your pocket!" he yelled and pointed.

"You don't see it, do you?"

"No!"

"Then I made it disappear. I didn't say I'd make it reappear, did I?" After loud protests, I said, "What's the magic word?"

"Please!"

"Please!"

I handed each boy back his own bill. Applause, applause.

Well, all good shows must end. John and Pop came to Mom's late Saturday morning, ready to head back to Garland. We got my car loaded, Charlie and I followed them home—and John didn't get lost even once.

Tuesday, July 18:

Further Adventures in Pop-land

One of Pop's hearing aids wasn't working—again—so yesterday I took it to Miracle Ear. Turns out it was clogged with ear wax—again. He's supposed to clean them first thing in the morning; the wax hardens overnight and can be removed more easily then, but he forgets.

George the tech chastised me. Hmph. Like I can control whether Pop cleans them or not. After the cleaning and lecturing was finished, I detoured to a dollar store and bought bags of birdseed.

Pop loves bird-watching from Mayberry's porch. He's been feeding the feathered flyers with leftover bread and has them so spoiled they raise a ruckus when they see him coming out the front door. He flings so much he ran out of stale bread, then got caught raiding the freezer for fresh bread.

He beamed when I carted in all those bags of seed. We made plans to look for a covered storage bucket he could leave on the porch, because carrying an open bag of bird seed while trying to manipulate a walker probably isn't the best of ideas.

Pop said he had some swelling in his lower abdomen. He very carefully exposed that area to show me what he was talking about. It looked like a waterbed sloshing around under the skin. He wasn't in any pain, but it seemed wise to have it checked out.

We saw Dr. A this morning, who asked some questions, slipped on a rubber glove, and told Pop to drop his drawers. I left the exam room.

What it *is* is a massive hernia Pop managed to give himself while we were in Tyler last week—probably trying to hoist himself out of his old, broken-down leather recliner. Dr. McCute said it might never cause a problem, but still referred us to a surgeon who specializes in such things.

Now lest you think we never have any fun, House 2 had a Dessert Social tonight. Families and friends could bring desserts—or not. I had planned to bake cookies, but wound up on the phone all afternoon trying to get some of Pop's business sorted out, and ran out of time. John bought a pecan pie on his way home—with every intention of making sure he and Pop got the largest portions. And they did.

John and I were the first (and almost only) relatives to attend the social. Things were pretty quiet until his cousin Mary Ann blew in. Her own dad died about a year ago, and she's adopted Pop. She's a tiny person physically but huge in animation, humor, and caring. She can leave people rather breathless with her rapid monologues, but she enlivens a room when she enters it.

She's also one of the reasons I'm going to hell. When we visited her last year, I brought along my frosted Lemon Cookies. She's a devout Catholic, and had given up sweets for Lent. True, I didn't know that, and she had intended to eat just one and save the rest—but she ate them all before the night was over. I make devilishly good cookies. (evil grin!)

Anyway, Mary Ann sat at one of the dining tables, and not only told stories that had us laughing, but got some of the ladies to tell stories from their lives.

When the party wound down, I helped Dianne gather up dirty dishes before John and I eased on down the road for home. He made sure we had the rest of the pecan pie with us.

Thursday, July 20:

Pop's MRI results

They're good! Dr. J, the physical medicine doctor, said the MRI showed no neck injuries that would prevent Pop from receiving physical therapy. She'll arrange for a therapist to work with him twice a week.

"Maybe you could get a pretty young woman therapist," I said, glancing at Pop. "Well, maybe not—he's surrounded by women at Mayberry. He might prefer a man therapist... Nah! Try for a pretty young woman." He blushed.

"Barbara..." he warned. Dr. J and I grinned at him. He grinned, too, but tried to hide it by ducking his head and shaking it.

He told Dr. J he's sleeping in bed again. He'd been sleeping in his recliner because the strain of sitting up to get out of bed hurt his neck. Even after he felt better, and even though we'd been urging him to use his new bed, he wouldn't. I think he was finding a form of security in sleeping in his old blue recliner—if he didn't use the bed, then he didn't live at Mayberry, and he'd be going home soon.

When we spent last weekend in Tyler, he, of course, slept in his old bed, so he must have rediscovered how comfortable it was to sleep lying down. He didn't say anything about it to us though.

When he revealed he'd been using his bed, I grinned big time. He saw me and once again shook his head, growling, "Dog-gone you, Barbara." Gotcha, Pop.

Monday, July 24:

Good News, Bad News

First, Pop had a good visit with an old friend yesterday, one he'd known since his Texas Instruments pre-retirement days. They kept company for about three hours.

Second, this afternoon we saw Dr. D, the hernia doctor. The bad news is Pop should have the surgery. The good news is the procedure should be relatively short and simple since it's been caught early. If he waits, the part of the intestine that's pooching out could eventually fold in on itself, shutting off its blood supply and killing part of the colon. Fixing that would be much more complicated, dangerous and painful.

Hernia surgery is "outpatient" now. Jeez! Isn't everything? The doc will push the intestines back into place, then sew what looks like a mesh screen over the area to keep them from bulging out again.

The surgery hasn't been scheduled yet because Dr. D goes on vacation next week. My mom will soon be having her second cataract surgery. In addition, our local stamping store is having their storewide sale on August 1, at which I plan to buy lots of stuff that I don't know what to do with, and don't have time to use anyway. Since I want to be present at all three events, I hope to do some appointment juggling to make sure that's possible.

Meanwhile, tomorrow I'm meeting Mary Ann (remember John's first cousin from the Dessert Social?) for coffee. She found some childhood snapshots of John to show me. Since she didn't say anything about bringing a stack of unmarked twenties, I'm assuming they're as innocent as John always claims he still is.

Uh-huh.

Tuesday, July 25:

3 Bubbas and a PT

Monica, the Physical Therapist, is young, energetic and personable, while still being business-like and efficient. She's also "easy to look at" according to Pop. It's good I made a point of being there because she asked lots of questions he couldn't answer, plus she needed to see his insurance cards, which I now carry with me.

It took almost an hour to get all the forms filled out, and to do some basic testing of his strength and mobility. Monica told us the neck has three basic movements: up and down, side to side, and "ding-dong" (ear to shoulder, other ear to other shoulder). Pop has almost no ding-dong mobility.

After she left, I asked if he wanted to eat out—John would be home in fifteen minutes, and I wasn't about to try getting supper ready that quickly. Smooth-talking devil that he are, Pop grabbed his walker and said, "Let's go!"

We ate at Luby's Cafeteria again. It's easy, it's close, and John likes that I'm a cheap date. It costs less to feed me there than at a regular restaurant. Pop sat on our patio for awhile afterwards. When he was ready for John to take him back to Mayberry, Charlie and I followed them outside to say good-bye.

John opened the driver's-side door, then walked around to the passenger side to fold up the walker and put it in back. Charlie spotted that open door and jumped in while Pop was still pulling his legs inside the cab.

I started to call him out, but his anticipation over a ride was too funny. Then John got in. Charlie, squeezed in between two big men, looked just as happy as a dog could be.

A Kodak moment and I blew it. Nuts!

By the way, Pop called about ten last night. He'd just finished playing dominoes with Miss Bess and Dianne. Miss Bess whipped both their behinds. He was a little disgruntled that an "old woman" beat him at his game.

Thursday, July 27:
Sing along with Pop and the ladies

Monica waltzed in this afternoon to give Pop his first actual physical therapy session. She had him walk around the circular hall to get his blood pumping, then directed him through some simple neck movements—simple for me, not so simple for him. His neck could barely "ding" going to his right and couldn't "dong" at all to the left. He'd been so protective of the pain on his right side that the tendon had tightened up until it couldn't relax or stretch anymore.

Monica spent several minutes deep-massaging it—Pop groaned in pain. When she slowly pushed his head to the left, his neck actually bent. Wow! She worked on it again until he could tilt his head to the left a little bit on his own. I applauded and cheered! Pop looked proud. The tendon will tighten up again, of course, but if he'll practice his exercises every day, it should get better.

When I'd first arrived at Mayberry, a blonde lady wearing a spangly blue blouse was unloading lots of stuff from her car and carrying it into House 2. Turned out it was "Sing Along with Winona" day. As soon as Monica left, and even though we missed the first half, I asked Pop if he wanted to join the fun—like he had a choice as I steered him out his door and into the common area.

Winona was playing to a packed room. Ladies from all four houses had gathered in the living room, spilling over into the dining room to accommodate the wheel chairs. We found seats at one of the dining tables.

Winona comes to Mayberry once a month; she brings props appropriate to whichever holiday is closest—both Flag Day and the 4th of July in this case. All of the ladies sported stars-and-stripes hats and waved little American flags. Two ladies shook maracas, while a third jingled a strap of bells. Winona passed out large-print song sheets to aid failing eyes and memories. We sang along with Mitch Miller music playing on her portable stereo. She toodled her flute. The music was simply grand!

She also read news items about, or showed objects from, the early 1900s. Her genuine interest and enthusiasm inspired the ladies to talk about their personal experiences. They had lived those times and used those items. Pop spoke up three times to add his perspective.

Shortly after we joined the group, I snagged a flag-striped top hat for him. Winona handed me a sparkly red one. We waved our flags; she took our picture. When we sang, "I've Been Working on the Railroad," Pop switched to an engineer's cap and held onto an old caboose lantern. Winona took his picture again.

Miss Bess wore the assistant engineer's cap. Yeah, I know— you're thinking sex discrimination: Pop got to be engineer because he was the only male present. I think it's just because he had the only head big enough to fit the hat.

He had a good time. When I chair-danced to "In the Mood," he laughed, but I don't know how anyone can sit still while that number is playing.

Friday, August 4:

About Miss Kitty

We've been trying to find a home for her since May. We've contacted several rescue organizations, and wound up with a fiasco with the one group that responded. I filled out an adoption card at the local no-kill shelter, but they're full and have a long waiting list. John showed her picture around at work. We've asked everyone we know, done everything we could, and have had no luck placing her.

And as I've said, we certainly can't/won't turn her loose to fend for herself either here or in the country. It also wasn't fair to her, keeping her confined in a small cage, plus the boarding fees were really adding up. Something had to give.

In spite of Charlie's fear of cats, I went to the vet's one day with the intention of bringing Kitty home and keeping her in one room for awhile to see how she'd do, but she turned hostile on me. The staff can handle her, but I couldn't even get her out of the cage. I left without her.

Last night John and I reluctantly made "that" decision. I called the vet's office today and told them we'd be in tonight to say our good-byes to her. The office manager called me back a little later and said her daughter wanted to try keeping Kitty over the weekend.

Oh my god—a reprieve.

Pray if you pray. Otherwise cross your fingers and toes and hope hard. We don't want to tell Pop anything but that Miss Kitty was adopted.

Sunday, August 6:

Pop the goat

John flew to New York this afternoon for another four days of training sessions with his company, so last night we took his dad to a nearby Mexican restaurant for supper.

A lot of people develop sensitive stomachs as they get older. Not Pop. The man is a goat.

A waiter brought the standard tortilla chips and salsa dip—a small bowl for each of us. The salsa wasn't fiery hot but it wasn't exactly mild either. Pop loaded up his chips and finished his salsa almost before we ordered our meals. After the food arrived, he eyed John's dip.

"You gonna finish the rest of that, son?"

"Have at it, Pop." John slid his bowl over.

He emptied the rest of the dip over his tamales. I offered him mine, and he poured it over his rice and refried beans. The waiter noticed the empties and brought three more bowls. Pop poured every bit of each one over his food and ate it all. Never even broke a sweat. The man can still eat whole jalapeno peppers and glow only slightly in the dark.

He'd had his mouth all set for a pecan praline for dessert, but the basket by the register was empty. I told him there was ice cream at home, and he thought it sounded pretty good. Later, he sat out on the patio for awhile with John and Charlie. He demonstrated his neck exercises for us just to prove he's been doing them. The physical therapist keeps massaging his neck at the spot that hurts the most, and he's holding his head a little more upright.

After his meal settled enough for him to move again, we drove him back to Mayberry. It's funny. From the front I don't think he looks that old. But when we're all in the car and I'm sitting behind him, he looks old and small and fragile. He slouches down in the seat, though, so that makes him look smaller.

Pop doesn't sit upright if he can recline.

Tuesday, August 8:

Miss Kitty news

I called the vet's office yesterday morning to check on her. She was still with the office manager's daughter.

Miss Kitty has a new home!

We are so relieved and grateful…except tonight I had the unhappy task of telling Pop that his companion and fuzzy shield against loneliness had been adopted. He cried a little, but said, "I'm glad she doesn't have to stay in a cage anymore."

I had taken our recently acquired cell phone with me, having arranged for John to call from New York around seven. Pop and I were sitting on the front porch at Mayberry then, and he talked with his son not long after he got Miss Kitty's adoption news. At least that ended his evening on a high note.

Speaking of high notes, while he was talking with John, I went inside for a drink of water. Weird noises were coming from the second hallway, so I peeked around the corner.

That white-haired raisin Miss Frances, who had hip replacement years ago, and who moves forward about a foot a minute, Miss Frances—wearing only the tank top of her pajamas—was "dancing" in the hallway, rattling her walker, and shaking her naked little bottom in time to music only she could hear.

Flaunt it if you got it, folks.

Thursday, August 10:

Thursday with Pop

This morning, after I bought three pairs of jeans for Pop, I hijacked him: we went to the bank so he could get some money with which to buy my lunch—after we saw Dr. J. She mostly just talked with him—asked what kind of work he used to do, about his home in Tyler, about where he lived now, and about his emotional state.

"I'm the only man amongst nine women where I live," he told her with a sly grin. "I'm real popular." Made us laugh.

Dr. J had him move his head in different directions, then asked him to walk down the hall so she could see how his therapy was progressing. When he reached the far end, I quietly said, "Pop's been talking about getting another car. I'm not sure if he's serious, but he's a wreck waiting to happen. Please tell him he shouldn't drive anymore —ever."

Pop rejoined us, and we went back into the exam room. Dr. J gently told him that while he was improving, it was unlikely that he would ever gain enough mobility in his neck to make it safe for him to drive, especially since his reflexes were slow, too.

He accepted the verdict since it came from a doctor, but I think it made him sad. Me, too. Really.

He needed a haircut. We headed for the last place I'd had mine cut, but I turned left at the intersection, even knowing the shop was to our right. I made a rude comment. Pop laughed. He's getting used to my creative ways of reaching a destination. Hey, at least I'm usually in the general vicinity of—somewhere. I circled back.

"How would he like it cut?" the stylist asked me. What? Pop's not a kid; and he's not senile.

"It's *his* hair—ask *him*," I said.

After he got his ears lifted, we went to the hearing aid store at the mall to find out why his right hearing aid wasn't working. Broken volume control. They sent it off for repair.

"You ready to buy my lunch, Pop?"

"Why, sure!"

"Do you want to try a place in the Food Court while we're here, or do you want to go to a Mexican restaurant that's just up the road?"

He opted for the Food Court, even though we had to walk half the mall to get there. Took us awhile. Sometimes he moves along pretty well; other times he hardly seems to make any forward progress at all.

I don't think he really understood what the Food Court was about until he saw it. Raising his head enough to see the menu boards over the different booths was difficult enough; keeping it raised long enough to read a menu was impossible.

He decided he'd rather go to the Mexican place after all. He sat at a table near the entrance/exit while I brought the car around. It was straight up noon when we got to the restaurant. This is a very popular place, so having to wait only a short time before we got a booth was a pleasant surprise.

I have to say I don't care much for most Mexican food. Partly I think refried beans look disgusting; most of it just doesn't taste good to me. However, Mexican is what's popular in Texas. I can usually find something on the menu that won't gag me—like fajitas. The food isn't important to me—the company is.

The waiter brought the obligatory tortilla chips and one bowl of salsa dip. Pop scooped a chip and bit. I dipped. He double-dipped (dipping again after biting.) Then without a thought to what he was doing, he curled his hand around the bowl and pulled it closer, making it easier for him to scoop. He never looked up to see me grinning at him for hogging the dip.

I don't like to share after someone double-dips anyway, so when the waiter brought our drinks, I asked for another bowl. Just like that it appeared. Never before occurred to me to ask for my own— either they bring individual bowls or they don't.

Pop liked this place a lot better than the one we'd been to Saturday evening. He said it was more like the one he goes to in Tyler. Plus they had huge pecan pralines for sale at the register. He liked that, too.

He was ready to head back to the ranch after that. Rather than try to turn left across lunchtime traffic, I chose to turn right and go the long way around. When we finally reached a major intersection, I shook my head in disgust.

"I didn't know we were going to come out at this corner. I thought I was going in a different direction."

Crazy woman driver! I think I scared him. And he's the one who shouldn't drive anymore?

We were actually on the street that leads directly to Mayberry—I just didn't expect it to be. And for a change, I managed to make the left turn into their parking lot without cruising past it as I'm prone to do when coming from that direction. I drew that fact to Pop's attention. He whooped!

He was ready for his chair and a nap, well fed and tired.

Monday, August 14:

Pop's off and so am I

I was not real thrilled to notice that the five people who arrived before us had also signed in for a 10 a.m. with Dr. H. I suppose when you have assistants doing most of the work, and you spend only a couple of minutes with each patient, you can arrange to have a dozen people scheduled for the same time spot. I know this happens a lot now, but I don't have to like it.

The good news is he took Pop off another glaucoma medication. He's down to one now. His eye pressure was so low and his optic nerves looked so good that the doctor again commented that he didn't think Pop had glaucoma. I asked if he was kidding. He wouldn't answer me directly—would only say that his pressure was in the teens, and there was no damage to the optic nerves.

I expressed dismay that he had been on three different eye medications for years. Was he misdiagnosed? Doc wouldn't give me a straight answer to that either—maybe because he knew the doctor Pop had been going to in Tyler. He'd only say that he'd recheck the pressure in two months. If it was still down, he'd take him off the last drops and see what happened.

Glaucoma doesn't just go away, does it? Shoot—I know it doesn't. So what's going on?

Well, after we left the doctor's, we picked up a couple of prescriptions, went by the P.O. to mail a package, then stopped by my best friend Nan's place to drop off some stuff. She came out to the car and turned Pop's head with her flattery—that is, he turned it towards her so he wouldn't miss a word.

Still got him back to Mayberry in time for lunch. I went on home to get some things done before heading to Tyler tomorrow. My Mom's second cataract surgery is scheduled for early Wednesday morning. She didn't tell me I didn't need to be with her this time. She learns quick.

Wednesday, August 16:

Will they do the Third Eye next month?

Mom had cataract surgery on her left eye last month. She had the right eye done this morning. Will they do her Third Eye next month? Do Third Eyes even develop cataracts? Do some trees dance in the forest, flinging their boughs about in foliage abandon, only to trip over the roots of their more sedate neighbors and fall, which is why no one knows if they make a noise because all the other trees are laughing, which sounds exactly like leaves rustling in the wind?

But enough of my Far (out) Eastern philosophy. After Charlie and I made it to Mom's yesterday afternoon, I called John so he'd quit worrying about me wandering around in a forest somewhere, which would mean I really was lost, because I don't think there are any forests in east Texas.

Now that you're thoroughly confused, I'll go on with my story.

Mom's apartment is small: living room/office, tiny kitchen, bathroom about the size of the kitchen, and one bedroom with one twin bed—hers. *My* bed was an air mattress inflated to somewhere between flat and flatter.

The only place it would fit was on a strip of floor between her desk and a bookcase, which put my head at the kitchen entrance and my feet near the front door. In case of fire, Mom would have to trample over me on her way out the door, undoubtedly leaving me in the same condition as the air mattress.

I'm not un-used to a bed on the floor, but lack of cushioning wasn't the only reason I didn't get a lot of sleep last night. Just as I started to doze off, the refrigerator motor roared on near my ears, sounding like a vacuum cleaner. Mom's bed frame creaked whenever she shifted. The air conditioner blasted on, which set the ceramic chimes hanging over the front door to tinkling. Then there was the tinkling of the toilet tank leaking, me getting up to tinkle in the toilet, and the tinkling of the tags on Charlie's collar which I didn't dare take off in case he had to go outside to tinkle, which he did at 4:30 a.m.

Mom got up at 4:30 to tinkle, too. Only she tinkled inside while Charlie tinkled outside.

So it wasn't real hard getting up at 5:30 because I sort of already was.

They called Mom in shortly after we got to the eye center. They numbed her eye, popped out the old lens, popped in the new, wheeled her out, sat her up, gave her orange juice, and gave her instructions and stuff to take home—just like the last time. We were out of there in just over an hour.

I walked Charlie after we got back to her apartment—he hadn't been there, done "that" yet. Unfortunately we went farther than I

46

intended because I have less sense than the dog. I should know better. It got hot fast, and it was so humid, moisture condensed on the road. Charlie shifted into slow mode. My blood sugar started crashing—too much coffee in the waiting room, too little food. I was sweating more from the "sugar-shakes" than the heat.

My legs got wobbly, and I barely made it back to Mom's. I grabbed a can of one of those meal replacement drinks she keeps on hand and chugged it. Since they're mostly sugar, I started feeling better in just a few minutes. Usually I have a snack bar in my pocket when I walk Charlie, just in case, but like I said, I hadn't planned on being gone that long.

We later went out to get Mom a haircut, which she doesn't like, and to the grocery store. We have big plans for tomorrow, but I think we're going to stay in the rest of today. She did, after all, just have surgery.

By the way, Mom and I researched cataract surgery on the Internet tonight—rather belatedly since the deed is already done. We learned it's done by phacoemulsification. Essentially, a laser or ultrasound is used to fragment the cloudy lens inside its holding-capsule, the pieces are sucked out, then the silicone replacement lens is folded like a taco and slipped inside the capsule, where it unfolds automatically and helps itself to some salsa dip.

They don't even have to use stitches because the incision is so tiny—but they better keep Pop away from that salsa.

Saturday, August 19:
Cataracts and hernias

Mom had an early morning post-surgery check-up on Thursday, after which we browsed two used-book stores, had lunch, then went back to her place and spent the rest of the day talking and half the evening playing games. Too much stimulation and too much coffee meant I wound up getting to "bed" later than usual.

Mom disturbed me about 3:30 a.m. when she used the bathroom. Charlie wanted to go out about four but didn't do anything. I'd barely pulled the sheet back over me than he wanted to go out again. Still nothing. By then Mom was up once again and prowling, wanting something to eat, wanting to read her newspaper, but unable to get to it because I was blocking the front door.

I staggered back to her room and crawled into her bed—where Charlie woke me up again about six. If he didn't pee that time, I was going to wring it out of him. I was just a wee-wee bit cranky by then.

Oh, well, we wanted to get up early Friday anyway so we could do some yard sale-ing before the day set itself to broil.

Mom, who passed her bad sense of direction on to me, had written down addresses from ads in the paper. Remember, she just had eye surgery, so that may explain part of her piloting problems—which started the minute she had me turn the wrong way out of her parking lot. We took a map, but frankly, she stinks as a navigator.

We saw more of Tyler than we'd planned on seeing—and saw some of it several times since I tend to travel in circles. Eventually we found our way back to her apartment, laughing about how pathetic even our combined directional senses were. We didn't find much of anything good at the sales we stumbled upon either.

Meanwhile, back in Garland, John took his dad to the hospital on Friday, where it took a totally ridiculous five hours to process Pop's paperwork, and to perform a chest x-ray and EKG prior to his upcoming hernia surgery. I gotta tell ya, I'm glad I was out of town, and it was John doing it, not me.

After they escaped the hospital, they grabbed some burgers, then packed up and headed for Tyler. They planned to attend the annual memorial service at an old country cemetery located between Tyler and Whitehouse. Pop's wife and parents are buried there.

It's an outdoor service that starts late morning on the third Saturday in August—in Texas, where the "s" stands for "swelter." It makes no sense to have it when it's so miserably hot until you know that Tyler used to be a farming community. Mid-August fell between planting and harvesting, which allowed farm families to gather at the cemetery, pay their respects to the dead, then get reacquainted with the living. It used to be an all-day social event, but now it generally lasts only a couple of hours.

That's why Pop wanted his surgery scheduled for after the memorial—so he could see people he hadn't seen since before his accident.

John called when they got to Tyler, but we didn't get together until Saturday afternoon. The plan was for me and Charlie to follow them back to Garland. I've gotten pretty good at finding my way to Tyler, but not so good at getting home. It's all backwards. If you have a tilt-a-whirl compass in your head like I do, you understand.

Now—can anyone tell me how two partially-deaf people can hear each other just fine—but everyone else has to shout and repeat themselves—and *still* not be heard or understood?

Here's the scene: John got to my mom's door first, said Hi; started carrying my stuff out to my car. Pop, who had been slowly making his way up the sidewalk all that time, finally reached the door. I spoke to him, repeated myself twice, and when he still couldn't understand me, he turned to John (who was already back from the car) to ask him what I'd said—and then John had to repeat himself twice.

Pop's only working hearing aid was squealing. He kept taking it out of his ear to adjust it but turned the volume knob the wrong way, so it continued its high-pitched, nerve-grating whine, which made me want to kill something. We finally got him to leave it in his ear and turn the knob the right way—away from your nose, Pop, away from your nose.

Mom will wear only one hearing aid at a time, and that one is about fourteen years old and barely works. She says she can hear fine with it. She can't. She'll give the appearance of hearing me, then say, "Whaaaat?" Or I'll ask if her hearing aid is in, and she'll say she can hear me without it. Arrggghhh! "No, you can't, Mom!"

OK, so now you know that, in spite of my heavenly Internet screen name—StFlossie—I don't have the patience of a saint.

Pop came into Mom's apartment and sat. John and I carried more stuff out to my car. When we returned, those two were talking normally and hearing each other with no problem. *How* was that possible?

Anyway, we finished loading my car and got on the road. We arrived back in Garland late this afternoon. John, in an attempt to not set the alarm for too early Monday morning, wondered if it wouldn't be easier to have his dad stay with us Sunday night since we had to have him at Out-Patient Surgery by 6:30 a.m.

I told him that it might be a little easier, but I wanted Sunday for us. I'd been gone a week, for pete's sake. I wanted to sleep in my own bed again for two nights before Pop came here to recuperate.

John, being the smart man he is, saw how tired and cranky I was, and decided easier wasn't always the best way.

Tuesday, August 22:

Hernia surgery

Pop was already up when we called him yesterday morning, and was waiting on the porch when we drove up. Since it's a short drive to the Garland hospital, we made it to the out-patient surgery doors right on time—but they were locked. We sat in the nearby waiting room, waiting to be called in ... and waited (while the few hospital personnel we saw ignored us) ... and waited some more. We finally checked the doors again and found them unlocked.

"They" said we were late. "They" said they'd called Pop's name. "In what hospital and what waiting room?" we wanted to know. We weren't real happy with "they." Anyway, he stripped behind a curtained-off area before the nurses prepped him.

The anesthesiologist did a spinal; actual surgery took about an hour; no problems. Pop stayed in recovery for awhile, then they rolled him into the post-op ward to wait for the spinal to wear off. They said he could leave as soon as he could stand up and pee.

While we were waiting for some action, Pop was, of course, just lying there, relaxed, half-dozing. Since John couldn't prowl around, he was bored. He noticed some coarse hairs near his dad's right ear, pulled out his trusty Swiss army knife, extracted the tweezers and started plucking. Pop didn't react until John plucked one hair in a particularly sensitive spot, then he jerked and yelped, "Oh damn!"

He had IV's in his hands, he'd just had his gut cut open—and it was a little plucked hair that made him almost levitate out of bed.

I couldn't help it. I started laughing, which got John started, which got Pop laughing, making him grab at his bandaged incision. He told me not to make him laugh.

Well, ultimately, he didn't have to pee for about seven hours. We dosed him with liquid. He dozed. We gave him more liquid. He dozed. John peed. I peed. John went home to let Charlie out and he peed. More liquids. John peed several more times. I peed again. Pop dozed. Finally we made him get up to at least try. He peed a little. We cheered, the nurses celebrated, and he was discharged at last.

He peed a lot after we got him back to our place.

He got up once last night, confused about when he'd had his surgery and what day it was. But except for soreness, he says he feels pretty good this morning. Mostly he's been sitting in John's recliner, watching TV and/or sleeping.

He has that male "remote control syndrome"—flip flip flip. Problem is, he doesn't always aim it accurately, and when it doesn't work, he starts pressing other buttons, which is when I hear the static, meaning he's turned off the VCR, and since reception comes through the cable via the VCR, the TV stops working. After I press the right buttons and get the picture back, Pop is happy and dozes off again.

Oh, last night when he was walking from the bedroom to the living room, I was standing off to one side to steady him if he needed it. He reached out and put his arm around my shoulders and hugged me, telling me how much he appreciated all I was doing for him. Took me by surprise, but sure made me feel good.

Friday, August 25:

The post-op patient

The doctor said Pop could sit up for a couple of hours at a time, then he was supposed to lie down for awhile. That wasn't a problem Monday since he mostly slept.

Tuesday he stirred around a little more. He not only walked in the backyard, but he made the circuit of the house—a real challenge because he has to maneuver his walker around furniture and through narrow passageways. It's a lot of fun when he suddenly realizes he needs to use the bathroom and has to negotiate the maze quickly.

Periodically I would suggest he go lie down on the bed. He was fine with that, although sometimes he'd ask, "Is it OK if I get up in an hour?" Of course. And he was up in an hour.

Well, about 9:30 last night he dozed off in John's chair.

"Pop!" His head jerked up.

"Whut?"

"I think it's time for you to go to bed. You're falling asleep in the chair."

"No, I'm not."

"Yes, you are." He'd been up for about three hours and really needed to go lie down.

I insisted. He protested. I still insisted.

He got mad—and I mean he was furious. He scowled so hard his eyebrows almost touched his nose. When he pressed his lips together, the whole bottom of his face disappeared—he had taken out

51

his upper dentures earlier. He grabbed his walker and hurled himself out of the chair—as much as he could hurl.

He can't stomp his feet anymore, but he can sure stomp that walker. He flung it sideways to move between the TV and an end table, narrowly missing the TV screen. And as he swung the walker into the hall, one wheel hit the wall. I'd been following behind to make sure he didn't tilt backward while he was flinging.

"I know you're angry, but you don't have to wreck the house."

He turned and immediately apologized, all contrite. "It's OK, Pop." He apologized at least three more times. When John went back to our bedroom to check on him a few minutes later, Pop asked if I was still angry with him. John assured him I wasn't.

I never was mad, but I was really tired. I wanted to be able to unhook my bra, sit down and relax for a while before getting ready for non-bed (the couch.)

When you take care of someone, it's hard not to act like a parent, and even though I thought he needed to go to bed, I later told him I was sorry I'd treated him like a child.

He felt well enough Wednesday to go back to Mayberry. Got him settled, then I went to Miracle Ear to get his repaired hearing aid, and had the other one cleaned out. After he inserted them, he could hear me whispering because they were both working so fine.

I ran some errands, went home and cleaned my house—which hadn't been done in almost two weeks because I hadn't been there most of the time, then washed the bed linens in anticipation of sleeping in my bed again.

I went to see Pop Thursday evening. He seemed shaky, out of sorts, and tired. He'd been sitting up too much, and I think he was hurting more than he wanted to admit. Regulations governing assisted living homes don't allow employees to hand out medicines from a prescription bottle. They have to be dosed out from the resident's personal medicine box which is filled by the family. If he had asked for a pain pill, Dianne could have given him the bottle and he could have taken one himself, but he didn't.

I finally realized that maybe he didn't know he could ask for them, so I put his pain pills in with his breakfast and after-supper medications, enough to last him through Sunday. That should help him feel better during the day and help him to rest at night.

Dianne told me that all the ladies had been asking about Pop while he was gone, and they've been fussing over him since he got back. The man is spoiled. And he loves it.

Thursday, August 31:
Pop had one of those days

However, let's start with my morning. After walking Charlie, I headed out to have two new front tires put on the Dodge, thinking, "It's the end of the month, people haven't been paid yet, it's still early—maybe it won't be that busy." Unfortunately other people must have been thinking the same thing. Tire Man guesstimated it'd be two hours before they could get to me.

Hope for fast service, but come prepared to wait: I had three stamping magazines and a book with me.

All of the waiting-area chairs along one inside wall were taken. I looked at the few remaining empty seats lined up against the east-facing window-wall, sunlight pouring in, already over 90 degrees outside, and thought to myself: "Ain't no way I'm sitting by the window and baking. *Poppin' Fresh* I'm not."

I grabbed a warm chair, carried it over to a tire display on the other side of the room—in the shade—plopped myself down, used one of the tires for a foot rest, and started reading. No one chastised me for making myself at home. In fact, it was so cozy, I had to fight nodding off.

After the new tires were on the car, I dashed over to Petco to get the poor dog a bone—our cupboards were bare. When I realized it was getting close to time to pick up Pop for his hernia doctor's appointment, I hurried home, unloaded the bones, let Charlie out, grabbed a piece of bread and peanut butter since I was starving, then because the Dodge needed a front end alignment so the new tires would be happy, I called the car shop to be sure someone could drive me home because I didn't have time to walk back—and it was too hot anyway—but they couldn't understand "calgrem didids baarag" because you can't talk clearly with a mouthful of peanut butter. Man! I didn't think that sentence was ever going to end.

So here's another one: I dashed over there in the Dodge, dashed (slowly) home again with the older-than-dirt father of the shop owner—he moves the vehicles in and out of the bays—but I sure wish he wasn't driving any of ours because not only is he pretzeled-up to where he can barely see over a dashboard, but he starts our stick-shift truck in second gear (cringe cringe). The Pretzel drove the Dodge back to the shop. I got in the Olds and dashed over to Mayberry to pick up Pop.

He wasn't ready. I'd forgotten to call to let him know I was on my way. While I waited in the dining room, I talked with Margaret, Dianne's mother. She helps the residents with their baths—even Pop.

He does his own "lap dance," so to speak, under a towel across his lap, but she scrubs everything else. Except this morning, according to her, they argued a little, then he flat refused to take one. As I've said, Pop can't stomp, but he can sure put his foot down when he wants to.

He came out of his room at last. We weren't even out of the house before he started crying. He said he wished he could just go to sleep and not wake up; he felt like such a bother to us. He cried off and on all the way to the doctor's. Post-op depression?

Well, after all that rushing, we had to wait forty-five minutes for the hernia doctor, just so he could spend about three minutes with Pop to tell him there was some swelling around his incision but that was normal, that we could take the surgical tape off on Saturday or Sunday, now go and don't darken his doorway again unless he had a problem.

I mentioned Pop's depression, but he's a gut specialist. He doesn't do antidepressants; told me to talk to Dr. A. My pleasure!

Pop was feeling so bad I didn't have the heart to take him straight back to Mayberry. I asked if he minded if we stopped at the bank, which he didn't, so we did. Then I asked if he wanted to go to Walmart since he needed a few things. He said "Sure." He wouldn't ever go with me before (afraid of slowing me down), so this was good.

We got him a cartload of necessities: a package of razor blade refills, a package of bar soap (he doesn't like using the liquid soap Mayberry provides), three boxes of Little Debbie brownies (he loves them), two canisters of barbecue Pringles, two packages of Nabisco Fig Newtons, and two jars of dry roasted peanuts. It's not like Mayberry doesn't provide snacks, but a fella needs his own personal munchies.

By the time we left Walmart, it was almost time for John to be leaving work. I said, "How about if I call John and tell him he's taking us out to dinner?"

Pop laughed. Yeah! He liked that idea. So, back at home, I called John to tell him The Plan. We decided to meet at a Mexican restaurant that was more or less on his way home. I called Mayberry to let them know Pop wouldn't be there for supper.

John beat us to the restaurant and was already seated at a table, working on the tortilla chips and a large bowl of salsa. As soon as I saw it, I immediately—even before sitting down—asked the waiter/manager for two more bowls.

Predictably, Pop pulled his bowl in close, right to the edge of the table, tipped it for easier scooping. He must have pressed down too hard. It slipped off the table, flipped, and spewed salsa everywhere.

The men didn't move except to raise their arms, apparently trying to comprehend what happened. Well, Pop *did* say "Oh, shit!" immediately. As soon as the salsa hit the shinola, I was up and halfway across the floor, got the waiter/manager's attention and asked for help before returning to the table to find Pop scooted back, just starting to wipe off his lap with a napkin.

He moved his chair again so he could stand without stepping in the salsa. I wiped off the tops of his shoes. John scraped off his jeans. We got him seated on a different chair while Tall Cute Man-ager helped clean up the mess on the floor.

Brave Man then asked if we wanted more salsa. "Sure!" I smiled brightly. Pop poured two bowls of it over his meal, so it didn't go to waste.

We finished eating without further incident—or accidents. I boxed up the rest of my fajita chicken for the starving and neglected dog; we left the Sweet Thang a good tip, and headed for home.

Pop drove back with me—always leave with the date what brung ya. We'd left his Walmart stash at our house, because you can't leave snacks in a car when it's 106 outside (and 206 inside the car) without meltdown.

I pulled into our driveway, which slopes steeply enough to thrill the neighborhood skateboarders. Pop asked me to run inside and get his snacks, but then decided he needed to use the bathroom. I went around the car to get his walker from the backseat, closed that door, set the walker down where he could grab it, and moved around to the front of his door to keep it from falling back on him as he got out.

He stood and shifted to the side. Instead of letting me close the door, he grabbed the top of it, pulled it backward—and forgot to let go.

It shut on his little finger. Ow. (That's a condensation of the sounds he made.) He actually did some dance steps!

I pulled the door open again. His finger was dented and bleeding. He was in pain *and* he had to pee. Poor Pop. I dug a clean Kleenex out of my purse and wrapped it around his finger to keep him from bleeding all over everything, then helped him to the front door—where Charlie was so glad to see us (he could smell the chicken), he wouldn't get out of the way.

John, in the meantime, had pulled in behind us and—before I even turned off my car engine—had rushed into the house to use the bathroom. He missed the whole show.

Well, Pop used the bathroom—urgent things first—after which I bandaged him up. John took him back to Mayberry.

We saw Dr. J, the physical therapy doctor today. She asked how they treated him at Mayberry, asked about his surgery, then asked if there was anything more she could do for him. Pop started crying, saying he wished he could die.

"It's ironic," I said. "The better he feels physically, the more depressed he becomes." She said it's probably because he's more aware of what he's lost.

Pop's been on Zoloft since Mother Pat died, but I cut his dose in half about three years ago because it was causing severe memory loss and confusion—something his "geriatric specialist" in Tyler never seemed to notice. It's difficult to find an antidepressant for people over sixty-five because the side effects can be more pronounced. Dr. J will consult with Dr. A about it anyway.

She decided Pop's neck had improved to where he didn't need to see her again, although the physical therapist will come twice more. I told her that we'd been to a lot of doctors in the last four months, but she was one I'd miss. I appreciated that she never seemed in a hurry to get to the next patient, and she really seemed to care. Pop seconded that, and she gave him a hug.

We went straight back to Mayberry this time. He opted to stay in the living room where three of the ladies were watching a talk show. Better for him to be in good company than alone in his room.

Tuesday, September 12:
Social butterfly and dental patient

When Pop first moved to Mayberry, Elveena and Rob were sharing a corner room. Elveena moved to a nursing home last month; Rob went with her—he wasn't about to be separated from her after sixty-plus years together.

Their daughter invited Pop and four of the ladies to their wedding anniversary celebration dinner on Saturday. The party-goers were picked up, and returned several hours later. Pop didn't provide a lot of details—just that he was glad to see Rob again, the house was nice, the food was good, and he enjoyed himself. Sometimes it's hard to believe he has the gift of gab—well, actually he has the gift of blarney, but that's not the same thing.

Yesterday we saw His Cuteness, Dr. A. He didn't think Pop was clinically depressed since he doesn't always feel bad. That's true. John and I hear about how he jokes around with the staff and the ladies at Mayberry. Dianne said residents often put on their worst face for family; if they seem happy, family might not visit as often.

Still, we have no doubt his depression is real. Maybe if we can get him involved in some activities, he'd feel better. We're going to leave him, as is, on the Zoloft for another month. If he gets worse, we'll try switching him to a different antidepressant.

Dr. A drew blood for a follow-up thyroid test. He also decided to take Pop off one of his blood pressure medications because his BP has been consistently low.

"You must be getting younger," I said. "First you go off two of your glaucoma medicines, and now this. You're just all backwards."

"Hmmm...do you think my hair will grow back?"

"Maybe so, Pop, maybe so."

On the way back to Mayberry I asked him to be thinking about things he'd like to do. John and I would help him as much as possible, but he had to tell us what interested him besides driving around and watching TV. He said he'd think on it. I walked him inside, then had to run since I was meeting my best friend Nan for Half-Price Books browsing and lunch.

Pop had mentioned he'd like a haircut. This morning we went to a different barber shop since he didn't much like the last one—too much styling, not enough cutting. After I helped him into the chair, the barber looked at me and asked, "How does he want his hair cut?"

"*I* don't know," I said, flinging my index finger toward Pop. "Ask him."

You may have noticed, as I have, that it's not unusual for people to assume Pop's senile because he's old and uses a walker. He never comments, so I don't know how he feels about it, but it bothers me. I joke about Dr. A's looks, but he treats Pop with respect—as did Dr. J—and I appreciate that a lot. Pop does, too, I'm sure.

After his haircut, we headed for the Senior Activity Center for the first time. I told him he might have to fight off the women since he looked So Fine. He paused for a second, gave me a sideways grin, and said, "You'll help me if they get to be a little too much for me, won't you, Barbara?"

"Sure, Pop. I'll beat them off with a stick if I have to."

"You just might have to," he preened.

I had picked up a Senior Center newsletter a few days ago, so I talked a little about all the programs, classes and trips they offered.

"A wood carving class is starting soon—would you like to learn to whittle?"

"I don't know," he said. "I think I'd rather diddle than whittle."

"Pop!" I'd have gotten away with my shocked exclamation if I hadn't laughed immediately afterwards.

We wandered around the center. Several men had gathered in one room to play dominoes, shoot pool, or just to watch the games. One man introduced himself, and talked with us for a couple of minutes. Across the hall a group of women played bridge. A country dance class was two-stepping at the far end of the building. Pop could watch and enjoy the music even if he couldn't dance.

Enough! We had to high-tail it to the dentist. Pop hadn't been to one in almost ten years. After he settled in the exam chair, I retreated to the waiting room with my new *RubberStampMadness*— and the coffee I'd begged off the receptionist.

Linda, the hygienist, took x-rays, cleaned his lower teeth, and consulted with Dr. B. He came out and asked me to join them. John and I have been going to him since forever; I knew from his grim expression that all was not well in Pop's mouth.

Specifically, his upper denture was cracked and worn out, he had three cavities, and x-rays showed abscesses had eaten out the roots of three bottom teeth. Plus he had a huge cyst on his lower jaw.

He ought to be in screaming, rabid pain, but he's not. There's no way to save the abscessed teeth—they'll have to come out—but his remaining lower teeth are solid and will easily anchor a bridge.

Pop doesn't have dental insurance, and it's going to cost about two thousand dollars just for Dr. B's portion—upper denture, temporary bridge, permanent bridge, and three fillings.

The temporary bridge will protect the gum line while it's healing, otherwise Pop wouldn't be able to chew, which would mean munchie deprivation, and we can't have *that*. It will take two weeks to make the bridge, which will be sent to and fitted by an oral surgeon after he does the extractions and removes the cyst.

When I re-explained all of this to Pop afterwards, I told him he had a choice. If he were in poor health, then frankly, because of his age, he probably shouldn't bother having the work done.

Fortunately, his health was good, but abscesses meant infection, and since infection could negatively affect his heart and all the rest of his body, he really should get his mouth fixed. He agreed with my assessment, but he's not looking forward to it—probably more because of the expense than the work itself.

Another good thing: It rained! After seventy-four days it decided to downpour just as we were leaving Dr. B's office. I had Pop wait under cover while I ran to the car to get the umbrella I'd so optimistically thrown onto the back seat three weeks ago.

We stopped at a hamburger joint for a late lunch. We'd never been there before, even though it's kitty-corner from Mayberry. He got the quarter-pounder, and it was almost too much for him to finish. As full as he was, he still thought maybe he'd have some of the dessert Gabriella had saved for him.

I took a rain check. My leftover chicken was calling Charlie's name, so I headed on home.

Thursday, September 14:

Pop goes to the rodeo

Texas Instruments sponsors a Retirees Reunion every year. Pop enjoys attending the function, and John usually accompanies him as his guest. This time the theme was "Rodeo."

They drove to the rodeo grounds in Mesquite early this morning. They listened to speeches by "some head mucky-mucks." They ate lunch. They got a kick out of the monkey riding on a dog's back. They enjoyed seeing a famous bull rider ride a bull. Since Pop and John are two expert bull-flingers themselves, they probably bonded with the man.

They had fun. The End.

Shoot, how am I supposed to work with that?

Since they didn't have any juicy stories I could pass on, I'll just dredge up an old one instead: Once upon a time, a couple of years ago, I answered the phone to hear Pop's irate, indignant and irritated voice telling me a sheriff's deputy had just come to his door and given him a ticket for littering. If he didn't pay the eighty dollar fine, they'd arrest him and take him to jail.

"*Did* you litter, Pop?" I asked. He got quiet. Since he lived out in the country, he didn't have trash pick-up service. Either he had to pay to use the city dump, or he'd use the dumpster at a nearby church—and yes, he sometimes threw trash bags out along a back road.

"Well, yeah," he admitted, "but there was other trash out there. No one saw me. How could they know it was me?"

"What was in the bag?"

"I don't know—garbage…some papers…"

"Papers with your name on them?"

More silence. Then he said, "Dang!" I tried, unsuccessfully, not to laugh.

"They got you dead to rights, Pop. There's no way you can talk your way out of this one."

"Bye," he said abruptly, but as he was hanging up, I could hear him grumbling to himself about the law threatening to put an old man in jail for littering.

He paid the fine, but he let the sheriff know what he thought about it, too. It's a wonder he wasn't thrown into jail anyway!

Tuesday, September 19:
Pop makes an impression—

And he makes an impression in more ways than one. I've heard that old shyster say, "You're my favorite" to different women on staff. He can't remember their names, but he schmoozes them all.

Miss Bess invited Pop and some of the ladies out for dinner next week. She asked him not to wear jeans because they'd be going to a fancy restaurant. Since he doesn't have any dressy clothes here, and even though he's bigger than his son, I took two of John's sports coats for him try on.

The black coat didn't fit at all. The gray didn't fit too badly— as long as he didn't button it, but he didn't have any pants that went with gray. We had to deal with that later, because we needed to get going.

He wanted some toiletries and more Little Debbie brownies, so we headed for Albertson's. He saw the Big Lots store next to it, and asked if we had time to look around before his dental appointment. Sure, why not. I parked midway between the two stores.

As we walked towards the grocery store, Pop spotted two pay phones. He cannot pass a newspaper machine or a pay phone without sticking his fingers into the coin return slot to check for change. Nothing in the first one. Nothing in the second either, but he pretended to slip something into his pocket before drawing out several coins.

"Look at that, Barbara," he crowed. "Do you believe I found all that money?"

"Not for a second," I said, grinning. He shook his head in mock dejection.

After we bought his groceries, we walked over to Big Lots. We were wandering the aisles when I spotted a display of baskets made with small—but real—corn cobs. I picked up one and asked Pop if he wanted it.

"That's nice, Barbara, but I don't believe I have a need for it."

"Well, I don't know," I said, sliding my arm across his shoulders and leaning in close. "You might be down home sometime and run out of toilet paper, and this basket would come in real handy."

As he caught on to my meaning, he raised his head and looked at me. A grin slid across his face before he laughed.

"You just might have a point there," he agreed. But he still didn't buy the basket.

We lingered too long in the aisles and had to hurry to the dentist's. Pop had been brooding about the cost—agreeing to have it done one minute, changing his mind the next. He called one night, and I heard John tell him, "You probably don't even realize how bad your mouth feels because you're so used to the pain."

I piped up. "Tell him if he won't have the abscesses taken care of, it's pointless to fill the cavities because what's left of his teeth will rot out, too." I don't think Pop appreciated it, but I was irritated with all his waffling.

Anyway, it took the technician almost a half hour to get her act together so she could make an impression of his teeth for the temporary bridge. By the time she finished, we were hungry and decided to stop at that burger place near Mayberry again.

He ordered the steak fingers basket this time. It came with fries, a bowl of gravy, and two pieces of buttered toast. The toast seemed a little much to me since the steak was breaded. I wouldn't have thought anybody would even eat it—or at least figured most people would start with the steak fingers.

Not Pop. He pulled the gravy bowl close to the edge of the table and started dipping the toast. It must be an East Texas country thing, reminiscent of biscuits and gravy, which he really likes. He never even glanced at the meat until he was done with what he considered the best part of the meal.

It's interesting to watch him. He doesn't eat fast, but his whole focus is on getting the food from plate to mouth. His physical coordination isn't very good, so that may be why he concentrates so hard. Even unfolding the several napkins he always uses takes complete concentration.

We finished eating, and as we walked back toward the car, we passed a pay phone. I "pulled a Pop" by feeling in the coin return and pretended to slip something into my pocket.

"What did you find?" he played along.

"Looked like a half dollar to me—might be a dollar though."

His eyes sparkled. "Woooo! Aren't you lucky."

"Yes," I said, looking at him, "I sure am."

I pointed to a small thrift store on the other side of the parking lot, and asked him if he wanted to go in. He does like to browse for a bargain—although sometimes he gets more—or less—than he bargained for. Years ago he picked up a hammer at a thrift store in Tyler and offered two dollars for it. "Sold," said the clerk. Pop thought he'd gotten a real deal—until later when he found the one-dollar price sticker on the handle. He still chuckles about that.

However, we didn't find anything interesting enough to buy in this store. I delivered Pop to Mayberry—and I suspect he took a nap not long after I left him.

Wednesday, September 20:
P.S. to Pop's impressive day

He must have been feeling let down after all the activity yesterday. He was back in his "I wish I'd go to sleep and not wake up" mode when John saw him tonight. The State Fair was coming up soon, John reminded him, and he didn't want to miss that. Then Thanksgiving was just around the corner, and after that was Christmas.

Doggone, it looked like he was just going to have to wait until after New Year's, because he was going to be too busy and wouldn't be able to work dying into his schedule before then.

Pop was laughing and feeling better by the time John left.

Monday, September 25:
Pop the popular

Rob's daughter left a message on our machine Friday, saying she'd invited Pop and a couple of the ladies to spend the afternoon with Rob and Elveena. She said he thought it'd be OK for him to go (like he needed our permission), but she didn't leave a phone number, so even if it wasn't OK, what could we do? He was gone for about four hours. No details from him—just that he enjoyed himself.

On Sunday afternoon John and I brought Pop and all the pants in his closet to our house. He tried on each pair and modeled them for me.

Men seem to have weird ideas about what fits. Doesn't matter if front pockets are pooched open; doesn't matter if love handles are squished into love shelves over the waistband; doesn't matter how high up the crotch rides—if the pants can be buttoned, snapped or zipped, they must fit. That's why I was supervising.

Out of ten pants, five could be zipped. Of those five, two were a little tighter than even Pop liked, and one was too snug to be decent. He's going to have to get Little Debbie her own pants soon, because they sure can't continue sharing the ones he wears now.

Since it's cooled off a little, we've been urging him to walk for exercise. Sometimes he tells us he has even when he hasn't—could be he thinks trying to shovel snow jobs over us is exercise enough. It's certainly more fun.

We finally managed to fit him into John's brown suit jacket and a pair of pants that he could still sit down in without popping out at the seams.

Tonight's the night Miss Bess and her daughter are taking him and the ladies out for an early dinner. I called him about four and asked if he was dressed and ready.

"Just about."

"I bet you look spiffy," I said.

"You're damn right I do!" he confirmed.

+++++

As I was writing the above, Pop called. They're already back from the restaurant. He said they went to a steak place where he ordered the roast beef. He also said he didn't really have to dress up after all. Some other man—Miss Bess's grandson?—went with them, and he wore jeans. Pop just out-spiffed him.

Tuesday, September 26:

Pop around town

Since breakfast at Mayberry is served at 8:15, and he had to be the oral surgeon's, at 8:45, Pop didn't have time to eat, but I promised him breakfast at Grandy's afterward. I brought the x-rays from Dr. B's for Dr. R to look at before he examined Pop.

Personally I don't care much for Dr. R. There's something about his superiority complex that annoys me, but he *is* a very good surgeon. He removed a cyst from John's sinus cavity several years ago and did a darned good job. I didn't like him then either (John did), but results count for something.

Dr. R agreed with Dr. B's assessment. The big white area just below the bottom front teeth was a cyst. He pulled down Pop's lower lip and showed me the swelling. Man, I don't know how he's managed to eat anything—must be like chewing around a ping pong ball.

Doc said he could clean out the cyst and do the three tooth extractions in about forty-five minutes. That surprised me, but I'm guessing there must be so little left to the tooth roots that they won't resist being pulled. The cyst tissue would be sent off for biopsy, but they're rarely cancerous.

At the check-out counter we picked a day to have the procedures done, then the clerk asked, "Is 9 a.m. all right?"

"Sure," I said.

Pop spoke up immediately. "Uhhh, Barbara? I won't be able to eat afterwards, will I? Can we change it so I can have breakfast first?"

"Oh! You're right. I'm glad you said something."

We changed it to 10:15, and that was OK with him. Pull all the teeth you want, but don't make him miss breakfast. When his stomach growled, he looked at the clerk and said, "Death by biscuits and gravy is the way I want to go—and I'm behind schedule." She smiled and shook her head, apparently not knowing how to respond.

We wasted no more time; Grandy's here we come. Pop selected his "ambrosia" from their clog-your-arteries wall-menu, then led the way to a booth, maneuvering his walker through an obstacle course of tight turns and too many tables. His steady stream of "Sorry …Pardon me" to his "hit and run" victims was interspersed with pithy expletives muttered under his breath. I followed behind with our loaded tray, trying not to laugh out loud.

We settled in a booth. Pop purred as he dug into his food—or maybe that was his still-growling stomach. Either way, he made short work of his meal. He wiped his mouth, leaned back, rubbed his belly, and belched. "Scuse me!" He gave me a sly glance, then tilted a bit to his left, and "belched" from the other end. He looked around— innocent as all get out—and said, "Who fired that shot?"

I almost sprayed coffee. Pop doesn't usually—deliberately— behave that way in front of me (unlike his son), so he must have felt pretty perky after eating his first "down home" food in a month. He grinned, pleased with his joke.

From there we went to Walmart. His old watch kept stopping, even though the battery had been replaced twice in one month; he bought a new one. After stocking up on Little Debbie brownies, he said he wanted to give Miss Bess a gift as thanks for dinner Monday night. Flowers seemed like a safe choice, but none of the cut flowers looked fresh. After we checked out, we went to Tom Thumb to pick up a prescription and looked in their flower department. He chose a potted plant with red blooms.

Even though he was getting tired, he wasn't ready to go back to Mayberry. He saw a dollar store across the street, and we crossed over to browse. I spotted an ice cream freezer near the front door.

"Want one, Pop?"

"Well, sure!"

The owner/clerk didn't seem real thrilled with the idea of an old man with a walker dripping an ice cream bar around his store. He offered Pop a chair behind the counter, but it would have been like trying to get into Grandy's—too many obstacles. A stack of plastic tables for children was near one wall; we moved over there. I helped him sit, using the stack as a bench. I sat down next to him, and we enjoyed our after-breakfast dessert.

Done, we wandered up and down the aisles. He didn't see much of interest until his eyes lit on the bin of rubber snakes. He pulled out a cobra, grinning so hard I thought his cheeks would break.

Pop delights in scaring the unwary with rubber snakes and huge, fuzzy black spiders—I've been only one in a long line of victims. Thankfully, all his faux-vermin were still in Tyler, but that's not why I put my foot down.

"NO!" I said. "Absolutely not! If you scare one of the old ladies at Mayberry, she might literally have a heart attack and die. And if you scare Dianne, she will beat you severely before she throws you out on the street. No, you cannot take that snake over there! No, No, No!"

Pop reluctantly dropped it back in the bin, allowing as how I was probably right. He bought a rake-like thing for retrieving items that roll under beds and chairs instead.

I know, I know—not nearly as much fun as a rubber snake. But what I didn't point out is what I'm sure Miss Bess would do if he scared *her*. That potted plant she was getting from him would undoubtedly be returned in a way he wouldn't appreciate.

Wednesday, September 27:
Pop gets ganged up on

As you know, we've been urging Pop to get some exercise. A few days ago he mentioned someone had donated an exercise bike to House 2. It was parked in the dining room.

"Hey, maybe you could ride that," I said.

"Maybe I could if someone would move it away from the wall," he groused, with no intention of ever getting on it.

I told you that to tell you this: Dianne said a new woman was helping to prepare and serve meals. Because Pop was in such a good mood last night, he'd been joking around with everyone. He and this new woman had been teasing each other all through supper.

The scene in the dining room began when New Woman asked him, "Did you move this chair?"

Pop, for whatever reason, got defensive and angry. He essentially said if the "damn exercise bike" wasn't in the way, he could get through the passageway to the table, and "No, I didn't move the damn chair."

New Woman tearfully reported to Dianne, who said Pop didn't hear well and most assuredly had misunderstood her. Meanwhile, he must have been frying under the hot, glaring eyes of the nine women seated around the two dining tables.

New Woman went back to Pop and apologized. He, in turn, profusely apologized to her, admitting he had misunderstood her "accusation." All was smoothed over.

He finished eating, and escaped to the front porch—he thought. Except Miss Bess followed him outside and lambasted him. "How *dare* you lose your temper like that and use those cuss words!"

He tried to excuse himself, saying he hadn't heard correctly, but Miss Bess didn't cut him any slack. "Then you should have kept your mouth shut."

Poor Pop. Nine women against one man. He never stood a chance. But he does contrite real well, so I think he's been forgiven.

Saturday, October 7:

Pop and Spike

Pop's been stuck at Mayberry all week because I've been working. He called a couple of times on Thursday, forlornly repeating my name to the answering machine. (He can't seem to get the hang of actually leaving a message.) I decided to give him something to look forward to. I called and conspired with him on The Great Escape Plan.

After work yesterday I picked him up and brought him home. While waiting for John to arrive, I saw Spike the Cat in our backyard. He lives next door, but spends a lot of his time over here, on one of our patio chairs.

Spike is tiny. When he first crawled through the chain-links of the fence, he was probably too young to have a cat smell, and for that reason, Charlie was only curious about him. Now Spike is the only cat he's not afraid of. They've actually started playing together! Charlie will bounce all around the kitten, knocking him down, which makes the little spitfire mad, so he flings himself at Charlie's legs, trying to chew on them while Charlie tries to dance away. It's really funny to see that big dog trying to dodge a little bitty kitty.

Since it hasn't been that long since Miss Kitty got adopted, I was a bit hesitant about bringing in Spike for fear of depressing Pop, but decided to take the chance. I made the formal introductions. His face radiated joy when I placed Spike on his lap. He smiled and laughed the whole time he petted him. He never said anything about Miss Kitty.

I put Spike back outside after John got home, and we drove to that Mexican place Pop liked. When the waiter set salsa dip on the table, it occurred to me that "salsa" is also Latin dance music. With as much of it as he packs away, no wonder he likes to shake his booty.

Now, back up to last Saturday for a minute: John went to Tyler to cut the grass—and to bring back all of Pop's dressy clothes.

Which brings us to Fashion Show #2. He tried on pants and sports coats. None of his pants fit anymore, and he could button only two of the jackets. He and Little Debbie are just doing too many slow dances together and not enough polkas.

After the show, I saw Spike out on the patio and brought him in for another visit. I wish we could see Pop's face light up like that more often.

Wednesday, October 11:
The tough old buzzard

Pop made sure he had a good breakfast before I picked him up yesterday morning. On the way over to the oral surgeon's, he asked me to refresh his memory.

"Barbara, did you tell me this is going to cost thirty thousand dollars?" Mercy! No wonder he kept changing his mind about having the work done.

"No, Pop. Dr. R's portion shouldn't cost more than a thousand all together." His relief was so great, he almost floated off the seat.

Dr. R pulled the three abscessed bottom teeth, cleaned out the cyst, and sewed up the gaping hole it left. When the wound finally stopped bleeding, they moved Pop to a bench in the small recovery alcove. He still had gauze stuffed into his mouth, and, of course he was the epitome of cliché, because every time he tried to say something, it sounded like he had a mouthful of—well, cotton.

Being the totally sympathetic person I am, I kept cracking up. Pop, however, got a little ticked off that no one could understand him.

The dental assistant gave us post-op instructions, and we left sometime around noon, with Pop's lower lip swelling up like he'd had too many collagen injections. We stopped at a supermarket to fill antibiotic and pain prescriptions, and got back to Mayberry while the ladies were still at the lunch tables.

"Do you want something to eat, Pop?" Do a hog wallow in the mud? Of course he was hungry. He needed to have something on his stomach anyway before he took a pain pill. I peeled the crispy breading off the fish, added some mashed potatoes to the plate, and took it into his room.

He managed to get a little food down, but his mouth was still numb and wouldn't cooperate. Frustrated, he gave up. I took the plate back to the kitchen, and returned to find him fingering the cyst stitches. Ack! He'd started the wound bleeding again. I stuffed gauze into his mouth to apply pressure and absorb the blood, then laughed at him some more when he tried to speak. He bit me.

No, he didn't. I ran home to get a cold compress for his chin and lip—didn't think to ask if they had one on the premises. When I returned, his door was ajar, but I knocked, pushed it open to find it dark inside, and flipped on the light. Pop almost levitated out of his chair. He had dozed off, and maybe he thought the Lord had come to get him.

I stuffed his heart back into his chest, helped him position the compress, gave him a kiss near his eyebrow, and left for work.

It was almost two by then, and the only reason I went in that late was to put finishing touches to things I'd started yesterday. The design center showroom had been remodeled, and the company owner was going to tour it on Friday. Mona, my boss, wanted everything just right before he arrived.

Mona commented to me that not everyone can do detail work—the little touches that pull things together and enhance their appearance
—and she appreciated that I could. Pulling things together is actually what the design center is all about. Buyers meet with the gallery designers to choose and coordinate the interiors of their new homes.

As for my job—I'm a former permanent part-time employee whose position was phased out, so I became unemployed, except I then became a temporary part-time employee who worked until they hired a full-time employee to do the same job I'd been doing but in an enlarged capacity—a job I wasn't willing to take on for a variety of reasons, with Pop being one. Only now I've become the permanent occasional part-time Special Projects Person—which means I do whatever needs to be done when it needs to be done.

I met John at Luby's afterwards, we ate, then we went to check on Pop. He looks like he's been in a boxing match—big bruise on his chin and swollen lip—but he can eat again in spite of that. He's a happy man.

Friday, October 13:

Pop and Mr. Bill

Last night I loaded Charlie in the truck and went to Mayberry to see how Pop was doing. We found him sitting on the front porch, enjoying the cool weather. His lip wasn't swollen any more, but the bruise still covered the center and left side of his chin.

He sounded pretty chipper, and he was glad to see Charlie— who in turn was glad to see "Grampy." Of course, once the greetings were finished, Charlie wanted to explore the grounds behind the houses. After he ran himself tired and thirsty, we detoured into House 3.

Mona's aunt, Miss Obed, lives there. She's a feisty, outspoken lady; I stop by occasionally to say Hi. She never remembers who I am, but she likes Charlie, and she's always happy to have visitors.

Unfortunately she's not doing well. Mona said she had fallen last week and was using a wheelchair now. We chatted awhile, then I gave her a gentle hug before Charlie and I took our leave. Except for occasional gatherings—like Winona's Sing Along—Mayberry residents tend not to mingle between the houses; I don't know why. But on our way out, the only man in House 3 happened by.

"Oh! Hello," I said, then proceeded to introduce myself, to tell him about Pop—who even now was sitting on the porch at House 2—and hoped they could meet sometime.

"Why not right now?" Mr. Bill bellowed. He turned around and beat me out the front door.

Charlie and I had to cut across the grass at a trot in order to get ahead of him and alert Pop, who managed to get to his feet just as Mr. Bill arrived. Try to picture this meeting of two men who once stood tall, but now were bent with age—two stooped-over men standing only the width of Pop's walker apart.

Mr. Bill stuck out his hand as he straightened up, lifted his head to look at Pop, introduced himself, bent back down. Pop shook hands, straightened up so he could lift his head to see Mr. Bill, gave his name —and slumped. Mr. Bill rose up, said he used to be a school teacher and football coach, and wilted. Pop raised up to say he used to be a farmer and machinist, and drooped to folded position.

Up, down, up, down…It was like watching a couple of ocean buoys rising and falling with the swells, bobbing up and down in a sea of seniors. It made me smile to watch them.

Mr. Bill issued an invitation to Pop to walk with him in the morning. Pop said maybe they could get together for a game of dominoes. They shook hands again, and Mr. Bill set sail.

It would be nice if they got together occasionally, seeing as how they're neighbors.

Friday, October 20:
Pop goes to the Texas State Fair

John scheduled a day of vacation because Pop told us he'd like to go to the State Fair. He anticipated the event all week, then called this morning and woke me up, saying he'd decided he'd better not go because he needed to use the restroom too often. He was afraid he'd wet himself.

"There are restrooms everywhere, Pop. We'll make sure you go every couple of hours whether you think you need to or not."

"Oh. Well, that sounds all right...but when I get tired, you can just leave me on a bench somewhere so I won't slow you down."

"We're not leaving you on a bench. We'll rent a wheelchair when we get there, so you'll ride most of the time—but maybe you can use your walker in some of the buildings."

"Oh. When did you say you're coming to get me?"

He was ready to roll, but John was still in bed, and I had to take Charlie for his walk. About ten minutes into it, a car backfired and spooked him. He wanted to go home. No, no, no, he hadn't "done" anything yet. A few minutes later it started sprinkling. Just great— that spooked him, too. I kept forging ahead, urging the chicken dog onward.

About thirty minutes later, it quit sprinkling, and he started enjoying himself. Forty-seven minutes after we started, he finally went "on empty" and we headed home. Even before we got to the fair I'd already been walking for an hour. Oh, my aching bunions. Maybe Pop and I could swap out riding in the wheelchair?

We picked him up. John, aka Mister "I know where it is and what I'm doing," who had looked at a map of the fairgrounds last night, who teases me about my talent for getting lost, became Mister "I can't find the parking lot." Well, he couldn't find the entrance near the wheelchair rental place; we wound up driving clear around the perimeter of Fair Park, which is no short drive.

Eventually he lucked out; we pulled into the area fenced-off for handicapped parking. John went on ahead to rent the wheelchair while Pop and I trailed after him. We rapidly discovered that the walker would not hang from the handles of the wheelchair, nor would it lie crosswise on the arms with Pop holding onto it—either we couldn't negotiate doorways or we would "kneecap" pedestrians. John carried it back to the car. Then we made the first of many, many restroom stops.

Poor Pop. Since John wasn't used to pushing a wheelchair, he didn't initially pay much attention to the roads and sidewalks, which are full of holes, cracks, ridges and angles. Not only did he immediately hit several "potholes," but headed straight for a curb.

Pop clenched the chair arms and yelled, "Don't go over the edge!" He muttered something not nice that made us laugh. He wound up hanging on for dear life several times, but at least we know he didn't sleep through the fair.

At times, I'd spell John and take a turn pushing. Once, as we rolled towards a tent we wanted to check out, I hit a chuckhole that stopped us dead. I backed up, steered to the right—and hit the hole next to it. By then I was laughing so hard I couldn't push at all, and Pop was again saying things it was just as well I couldn't understand. I backed up again, steered right once more, and managed to get us moving forward.

John has this tendency to speed-walk past exhibits and demonstrations—which means everything passed by Pop in a blur. I learned years ago that if I hung onto John's hand and walked at my pace, he would slow down enough that I could actually see things. So now I deliberately slowed way down, which forced John to do the same if he didn't want to lose me in the crowds—and he knew he'd better not.

Sometimes I bent down near Pop's eye-level to point out things that were above his direct line of vision. He got his Masonic ring cleaned. He tried a sample of hot salsa, and bought a jar of it. I squeezed a hand lotion sample into his dry hands. He tried a cappuccino coffee sample, but didn't like it. I got a great back massage with a hand-held gadget. John bought large slabs of fudge for the ladies at Mayberry.

We saw a dog show, two band performances and all kinds of exhibits. Neither man would go on any of the Midway rides with me—no sense of adventure.

In spite of all the exotic cuisine available at the Food Court, we ate Mexican food for lunch. Later we shared a huge soft pretzel and some lemonade on the Midway. And we each got a dipped-in-chocolate-and-chopped-nuts ice cream bar.

We parked Pop near the ice-cream stand so we could eat them before they melted. Some of the chocolate coating and several nut pieces landed on his shirt and in his lap. I got the chocolate off his shirt, but told him, "The nuts in your lap will fall off the next time you stand up to use the restroom."

"I *hope* not!"

John roared. Pop grinned, mightily pleased with his joke. It took me several seconds to figure out what was so funny.

Late that afternoon we finally steered back toward the parking lot. We made one more restroom stop, rolled Pop to the car, John returned the wheelchair, and we headed home—just about the time it stopped sprinkling and started serious raining.

Pop said he enjoyed himself, but suddenly became reflective and melancholic, musing almost to himself that he'd probably die before the next State Fair. John and I were stunned into silence.

The next moment he seemed to realize what he'd said, and apologized—declaring that of course he'd be going to a lot more fairs.

"You bet you will, Pop," I agreed, "and maybe next time I can get you on one of those Midway rides."

"Next time?" he snorted. "Wasn't I on one all day today?"

He had a point there.

Saturday, October 28:

Pop goes to Tyler

I wanted to go to a Tyler book fair with my mom, and that was as good an excuse as any for John to take more vacation time. He, Pop and Charlie would all enjoy some country time, too.

Mom and I shopped for books Thursday morning, and took care of items on her errand list. Meanwhile, back at the ranch, John broke both the riding mower and the push lawn mower while his dad supervised. Don't ask. I didn't.

When I went back to Pop's for the night, I had him soak his feet in a pan of water until his toenails softened up. They're so thick and tough, they're tearing up his socks—not even Dr. A was able to cut them. It was the first time I'd ever given a pedicure and the first time Pop received one. We were both grateful there was no bloody mess to clean up afterwards.

Early Friday morning Mom and I hit several yard sales, but didn't find much of anything. I called John when we were done. He and Pop came to her apartment to collect me and Charlie so we could head back to Garland together.

I'm OK when I leave from Pop's, but since I've seldom driven home from Mom's, getting out of town from her place is confusing to me. It seemed wise to follow the men, which I was doing—until John pulled off to the side at an intersection to wait for me to catch up. It wasn't the first time we'd ever done this because John seems to think speed limit signs are only a suggestion, and I don't.

Anyway, I breezed by the truck, knowing they'd catch up and bypass me so I could follow them again. When they didn't, I turned around expecting to find them back at the light. They weren't. Thinking I had somehow missed seeing them get in front of me, I turned around again.

I drove far enough that the scenery didn't look familiar and I still didn't see them, so I turned around once again, got back to the light and turned in what I thought was the right direction, drove until it seemed like the wrong direction, then turned around yet again.

Driving in circles is my specialty. My biggest concern was being lost long enough for it to get dark. I don't drive well in the dark. Mostly I can't see. Charlie, who was trying to sleep while I muttered dire threats of future bodily harm to John, made me feel less alone, but was no help otherwise. Eventually I got smart enough to pull into a gas station, got directions, and made it to the highway.

I caught up to them at the first rest stop. John was on a pay phone calling my mom to see if I'd wandered back to her place. He had also called my cell phone, but since I didn't answer, he thought I was mad at him. I was! He lost me! He's not supposed to lose me.

As mad as I was, I still would have answered my phone because I wanted him to tell me how to get found. When I'd finally noticed the voice mail indicating he'd called, I thought the phone hadn't rung because it wouldn't ring for incoming long distance, which made absolutely no sense, but I was a little stressed out by then, OK? It didn't matter anyway, because I couldn't figure out how to connect to the voice mail.

It was just as well we were in separate cars because I was really mad by that time—although if we hadn't been in separate cars, I wouldn't have gotten lost. Plus, I was just as mad at myself for being so dependent as I was mad at John for losing me. I could barely speak to him—partly because I didn't want to burst into tears. I still had to drive the rest of the way home, and I can't see when I'm crying any better than I can see in the dark.

Then John got mad at me for being mad at him—which made me even madder, if that were possible. How *dare* he get mad at me for being mad at him! Pop, who could tell I was furious, thought I was mad at him, which upset him. Charlie was the only one who felt good. He thinks rest stops are real interesting places.

Well, we finally made it to Garland. John took his dad back to Mayberry while I went on home. The first thing I noticed when I walked in was the "in use" light on our phone was lit. Ghosts? Picked up the receiver and heard nothing but noise. Who knows how long it had been like that.

I unplugged everything, waited, plugged it all back in. Noise. I walked next door, not only to get our mail—which our neighbors had picked up—but to borrow their phone to report our problem. It never occurred to me to use my cell phone.

After pressing all the buttons and listening to all the garbage— including the stupid suggestion that if I wanted to check the status of a reported problem, I could go to their website even though I couldn't go anywhere on the Internet because we're on dial-up and the darned phone wasn't working—I finally pressed a button that took me to Martha.

"Martha!" I gushed. "It's so nice to finally get a real person!"

"What seems to be the problem?" she asked, trying to be business-like.

"My phone broke," I wailed. "My life is over! Why do you think I'm calling you?"

She dropped her professional face and laughed. She asked a couple of questions, then told me what to do.

"Do you promise my phone will work after that?"

"Yes," she said.

"If it doesn't, is there some way I can reach you without going through all the press this and press that again?" Yes! She told me what to do and gave me her extension number.

Well, her instructions didn't solve the problem, so I called her back—on the cell phone this time. She said she'd done a second line-check after we'd hung up and knew it wasn't an inside-the-house problem, but she'd forgotten to ask for my neighbor's phone number and couldn't call me back. They sent out a phone repair man this morning; got it fixed up.

Oh yeah. Last night—after John and I were speaking to each other again—he said he'd seen me in his side-view mirror as I approached that first intersection, but had looked toward Pop just as I went by and didn't see me drive straight ahead. He'd assumed I'd turned left at the light like I was supposed to. No wonder he couldn't catch up to me.

When we compared notes, something didn't compute. He called my cell phone. It didn't ring. He tried again. It still didn't ring. The ringer was broken. What a headache.

Take two phones and call me in the morning.

Wednesday, November 1:

Pop does Walmart

This morning I took glaucoma eye drops and new socks over to Pop. I forgot it was bath day and arrived just as he was heading down the hall. Margaret, who helps the residents bathe, said he was wearing underpants under his wrap/tie robe—I assumed that was so he wouldn't "wave" at any of the ladies en route.

She asked if I'd seen his snap-front robe; neither of them could find it. He said he couldn't find his denture brush either. John had been in charge of packing up Pop's stuff before we left Tyler, which means that's probably where the robe and brush still are.

"Do you want to go to Walmart with me?" I asked. Yes. He'd felt blue yesterday and hadn't wanted to get out, but he was in a much better mood today. I went home and puttered around while waiting on His Cleanliness.

It was almost lunchtime before he was ready, but rather than eat at Mayberry, I suggested we eat out, either before or after we went to Walmart—or even in Walmart, for that matter. McDonald's had a concession stand inside. He decided he'd like to eat there, then shop.

He ordered a double cheeseburger and fries. I got him settled at a table, carried our food over, then went to the condiments table and grabbed a handful of what I thought were packets of ketchup, but turned out to be hot picante sauce.

"Hey, Pop—just what you like!" I tore one open for him; he squeezed it onto his burger. A few seconds later he started coughing.

"You all right?"

"THAT'S HOT!" he said, outraged.

I broke up. It must have been sizzling if it was too hot for him. I asked him a couple of minutes later if he wanted more sauce on his burger. He didn't even raise his head—just gave me "that" look over the top of his glasses. If I had cackled any harder, I'd have laid an egg.

While we were eating, he said the front and left side of his mouth was sore. The front I could understand—he'd just had that walnut-sized cyst removed. He doesn't usually complain about pain unless he's really hurting, and the left side of his face did look a little swollen. I said I'd call the oral surgeon from home.

On to shopping. Pop bought only the essentials: two bags of birdseed, a denture brush, three boxes of Little Debbie brownies, two cans of Pringles, a bag of chili cheese Fritos, a package of Fig Newtons, and a bag of fun-size Snickers. I can hear the man's arteries clogging from here.

After I dropped him and his groceries off at Mayberry, I called Dr. R's office. They said to bring him in at three. Oh, great—it was already after two. I called Pop and told him to be ready to go out again in fifteen minutes.

We rushed to Dr. R's—and had to wait. It was quiet and warm; Pop can be quite relaxing to sit next to. I was reading my *RubberStampMadness* magazine when I think I dozed off.

They finally called him into an exam room. Dr. R discovered a small pressure ulcer along the gum line where the temporary bridge didn't fit exactly right. No wonder it was sore. Pop said it felt much better after it was adjusted.

"Magic fingers," Dr. R said, waggling them at us. (OK, I gotta admit I like his sense of humor, superiority complex or not.)

I tell you what—Pop is a charmer. The three office ladies at Dr. R's told him he's sweet. The ladies at Mayberry like him and take care of him. Miss Bess smooches with him. The wild birds get all excited and make a racket when they see him come outside—they're probably females. The man even got me to let him buy three boxes of brownies instead of two, after I suggested he cut back on the snacks since his waistline had expanded.

Shoot, no wonder I married his son. John certainly inherited his dad's charm—but he still can't pack a suitcase worth a darn.

Wednesday, November 8:
Mayberry Stamping Party!

When I discovered rubberstamping, it fulfilled my craving for an artistic outlet. I can't draw or paint, but with ink pads in assorted colors, a few rubberstamps, and various kinds of cardstock, I create greeting cards. Not only do I illustrate the card fronts, but I like making up my own captions or silly verses for inside.

That information is for you non-stampers. Stamping is my joy —and I got to share it. I talked with Dianne about having a stamping party. She liked the idea, and we set a date—today.

When I mentioned it might be fun for the Mayberry ladies to make Christmas cards for their families, several people on my Rubberstampers List sent stamped images, cardstock, ribbons, stickers and other items for us to use. Stampers are some of the most generous people in the world.

When I hauled over the stamping supplies this afternoon, Miss Dorothy was sitting on the front porch. "We're going to make Christmas cards," I told her.

"I don't know how," she said.

"It's easy," I said, reassuring her. "It'll be fun."

We went inside. Miss Pearl rolled into the living room in her wheelchair. "We're going to make Christmas cards," I repeated. "Want to play with us?" Her eyes brightened, and she followed Miss Dorothy and me into the dining room. Dianne knocked on the doors to everyone's rooms to invite them to the party. Before long, Pop and six more ladies joined us.

I unpacked my shopping bags. In addition to the donated items, I'd also brought the fronts of old Christmas cards to reuse, holiday napkins, my camera, and a Xyron—a small, hand-cranked machine that quickly applies a thin layer of adhesive to one side of paper—much neater than glue sticks.

Pop and the ladies sat at the long, rectangular dining tables. It's funny. I suddenly got stage fright, seeing all those expectant faces turned toward me. What made me think I could teach them anything? Then Pop caught my eye and winked at me. I grinned at him, took a deep breath, and passed around three cards I'd made as samples.

"Any way you make a card is the right way." I told them. "You absolutely cannot do anything wrong." I emphasized this because they always seemed to be afraid of making mistakes. "You can decorate your cards with anything you want to—and anyway you want."

They were tentative at first, but we took it step by step. Dianne began by helping Miss Dorothy; I helped Pop. He had a choice of red, green or white cardstock. He chose red. Then he picked out a picture of a stained-glass window. I slipped a piece of silver paper between it and the cardstock. "What do you think?" I asked.

"It's nice—pretty," he said.

I ran the picture and silver paper through the Xyron, and helped him peel off the backing, He stuck them onto the card front, silver paper first, the stained glass window on top. He looked through the pre-stamped greetings and selected one. He ran the paper through the Xyron this time, and placed the sticky paper inside his card.

When he was done, I clapped and said, "Hold it up!"

He held up his card with a flourish and boasted, "See how easy that was?" He really made a big production out of it, which made the ladies smile.

Everyone finally relaxed and began playing with the materials, chatting while they sorted through the pictures and passed things to each other. Pop scooted his chair closer to Miss Bess and helped her pick out images.

Miss Helen made a card with a Santa cut-out. Miss Pearl liked both the laminated gold angels and another angel image, so she made two cards. Miss Frances picked out two puppy images and made two cards. Miss Dorothy glued a teddy bear napkin to her card front. Since the napkin also opened up like a card, I suggested she stick something inside it—then she had two cards in one. It was so cool that she held it up to show everyone how it worked.

Miss Lela fluttered her hands nervously. "I can't do this by myself."

"I'll help you," I said. She eventually picked a holly-print paper that she covered with green paper, then…well, she kept piling things on top of that. After she layered pictures and papers a half-inch high, she announced, "I'm done now," and turned the whole thing face down on the table.

Miss Clara also needed special attention. She was in the early stages of Alzheimer's disease and had trouble making decisions. She shuffled through pictures and cardstock over and over, fretting about what she should do. Dianne reduced her choices and helped her place images. She wound up making two cards and excitedly shoved them into her duster pocket.

A couple of hours later they all had one or two cards they proudly posed with while I took snapshots of them. I wanted to remember that day and those smiling faces. I do believe I had more fun than anyone else.

Sunday, November 12:

Catching up with Pop

This is kind of personal, so I'll try to be delicate: Pop has to pee a lot.

He'd been complaining about how often he has to get up at night, not to mention how often he has to go during the day. At almost 82, it's a pretty sure bet his prostate is enlarged again and causing the problem, but it needed to be peeked at just to be sure.

I called the urologist Pop went to when he first moved here, and asked the receptionist if he could he come in sooner than his scheduled mid-December appointment?

"Nope, absolutely not—no openings."

"What if this were an emergency?"

"Go to the emergency room."

I didn't like her attitude, and who needs a doctor who's too busy to see you? I got out the insurance provider directory, called some other doctors and found one who was able to see Pop on Friday.

I picked him up in what should have been plenty of time, but he had to make another pit stop before we left. Then he saw something in the parking lot and slowly bent down to pick it up to check it out. It must have taken fifteen minutes to walk the short distance from his room to the car, and then he had trouble getting into the car.

Pop is definitely teaching me to slow down. I'm always going at top speed until I'm with him, and then it's almost like I'm sliding backwards as snails zoom past us.

By the way, when we walk together, I frequently touch his back or arm. I believe touching helps people know they're alive and real, and it's especially true for people who live alone. Touch reconnects them to the world. Of course, the contact is brief, and I don't touch people who seem adverse to it. Shoot, I don't want some people touching me.

Anyway, since I wasn't sure exactly where the new urologist's office was, I initially parked at the wrong building, but was smart enough to run in by myself first to check the directory. When I didn't see the doctor's name, I dashed back to the car, drove a little further down the road and found the right building.

Pop peed in a cup, then Dr. U did the mandatory grope examination. No surprise the prostate was enlarged, but he also wanted to examine the bladder with a scope to make sure there weren't any other problems. We set up another appointment before Pop went down the hall to have blood drawn.

It was late by the time we got away; I brought him home with me. We convinced John that eating out was a good idea, especially since I hadn't fixed supper.

Moving on: Remember Pop's temporary bridge adjustment? Naturally, once you get one side adjusted, the other side goes awry. Now the right side of his mouth was sore. I called our dentist this time since I was pretty sure infection wasn't involved.

I picked up Pop, who was standing in his doorway, telling the lady who cleans his room where he was going. She gave him a big hug. That man sure gets a lot of sugar.

On to the dentist. Pop got settled in the exam chair. The dental assistant bent the bridge wires this way and that, and put it back in his mouth. He thought it felt better. We left. We were still in the parking space when he started popping the bridge out with his tongue, worrying at it, not sure if it felt right or not. We went back inside.

The DA fiddled and fuddled and muddled. She couldn't get the bridgework to sit without rocking. Another lady came in to observe and asked if she needed help. Dr. B stopped to say Hi, watched for a minute, then came in and took a look.

It seems Pop's gum line had changed since the surgery—like it was missing a big swollen cyst. Dr. B needed to build up the bridge to make it narrower in order for it to fit snugly, which took a while since he had to build, test, build, test. During the process he told me that cysts eat out the bone in order to make space for themselves as they grow. If Pop hadn't had it removed, one day he would have bitten down on something and his jaw would have shattered. Mercy!

Dr. B eventually had him all re-fitted and feeling better.

On Friday, Pop didn't mind running an errand to Half-Price Books before Dr. U's appointment. It took only five minutes to get and pay for the book, but Pop came in with me, and sat near the front of the store. Before we left, he had to use the restroom, which was clear at the back.

When he finally reappeared, he stopped near an alcove, turned to face into it, waved me away when I moved toward him, and adjusted his pants. When we got to the car, he concealed himself behind the open passenger door and adjusted whatever the problem was again. He seemed so disgusted with himself that I didn't ask what was wrong.

We drove clear across town, into Richardson and back toward Garland to get to the doctor's office—and actually made it with three minutes to spare. They called him in almost before we sat down. Nurse told him to pee in a cup, then take off his pants and underpants. Pop went into the adjoining restroom/changing room. It got real quiet after the flush. I finally asked him if he needed some help.

When he opened the restroom door, his shirt was unbuttoned, but he'd forgotten how much of his clothing he was supposed to take off. I repeated the nurse's instructions. To make it a little easier for him, I had him lean against the exam table while I took off his shoes, but told him he was on his own for the rest. When he started to unzip his pants, I headed out the door—just as the nurse came back in. She helped him get ready.

The actual scoping to look inside his bladder didn't take long. Without going into detail, there was a bit of blockage, but not enough to warrant surgery. The only thing that concerned the doc were the higher than normal levels of calcium in last week's blood test results.

Doc said this could indicate a malfunction of the parathyroid glands (near the thyroid), and could be caused by a variety of reasons, including cancer. He suggested re-testing, and if the second results were high, Pop should see his family doctor for further tests.

We stopped at the lab again on the way out. Since we were the only ones there, the fella who wields the needle asked Pop if he'd mind being stuck out in the waiting room, rather than trying to maneuver his walker into the lab room again.

"Do I have to take off my pants?" Pop asked me.

"Not unless you just want to." He started unbuckling his belt. I squealed. He and Fella laughed.

We headed back to Mayberry. When we were getting close, I asked Pop if he recognized where he was. He wasn't sure. I pointed out John's church, the barber shop he'd been to where the barber had manhandled him in an effort to help him into the chair, "and just a little further down the road is your home." That's the word I used.

"It's where I stay," Pop countered immediately. Home for him will always be Tyler.

Tuesday, November 21:
John broke the car—and smooching on Pop

We had planned on taking both cars to Tyler for Thanksgiving because there was no way we could load three adults, a dog, suitcases, and food (there's nothing at Pop's house) in just one vehicle.

However, the Dodge had started stalling at odd moments—like when it was moving. That's nerve-wracking enough in city driving, but if it stalled while going seventy on the highway, it would be more thrill than I could handle. John said he'd been praying about the problem.

Today he took the car to gas it up. He misjudged the turn into a gas station, hit the curb, and now there's a grinding noise under the front left fender. He wasn't going fast, so he must have hit at just the wrong angle. Anyway, the Dodge is in the shop. Be careful what you pray for. (grin)

The broken car means we'll be having Thanksgiving in our own home for the first time in twenty-nine years. John is going to Tyler tomorrow to get my mom so she can spend a couple of days with us, which will be fun.

Of course, it was fun last year, too, at Pop's house. I'd found an apron while I'd been doing some cleaning for him and decided to wear it because in my enthusiasm over doing dishes by hand, I have a tendency to splatter water and assorted food debris all over me.

Wearing an apron made me feel like June Cleaver, minus the heels, pearls and housedress. Well, it wasn't a frilly apron like hers, but a red-checked bib number imprinted with big black letters reading "HOT PANtS." Since it had belonged to Mother Pat, I was shocked. Mothers would *never* do "It"—although if you're wearing an apron minus the housedress, I could see how you might wind up with children.

84

After the meal, Mom helped put the food away, then she went down for a nap in the guest room. Pop retreated to his bedroom, too. Since the temperature was delightfully cool, John decided to take a walk. I started on the dishes.

So, there I was, in my not-frilly apron, thinking about how June must have begotten Wally and the Beaver, became interested in testing the apron theory in the privacy of one of the handy storage buildings—and no John anywhere in sight. Ah, well. When the dishes were done, I took Charlie for a walk instead.

Anyway, celebrating Thanksgiving at home in Garland this year meant I could start dinner preparations in my own kitchen, plus get some other stuff done before John and Mom got here. When John takes her home on Friday, he and Pop will spend the night in Tyler and return Saturday, which means while they're gone, I'll get even more stuff done—and isn't Thanksgiving all about stuff-ing? Thus, aside from the $$$$ it's going to cost to fix the Dodge, I have a lot of stuff to be grateful for.

Oh yeah, smooching on Pop: John's cousin Mary Ann brought her arsenal of cosmetic samples to Mayberry today. She spent the afternoon "painting" the ladies' faces, then someone else poofed their hair. I helped by telling them how pretty they looked. Mary Ann took their pictures, and will have 5x7s made so the ladies can give them to their families for Christmas.

After the individual glamour shots, Mary Ann had the ladies gather around Pop and snapped a group picture—he had come out of his room to watch the show when it was almost over. I tried to put some lipstick on him, but he wouldn't have any part of it.

"I'd rather wear my lipstick second hand," he said.

The old letch!

Monday, November 27:
Post-Thanksgiving Pop

Since we weren't going to Tyler, I called Dianne and asked if the ladies who weren't eating with their families would like to come here for dinner. She said the thirteen "leftovers" from all four houses were going to feast together in House 3. Thirteen is way too many for our dining table to seat, even if we had one, which we don't, because our dining nook is my office.

Shoot, if I'd been smart, I would have had Pop invite all of us to dinner at Mayberry. It would have saved me a lot of cooking and cleaning up, but where's the fun in that?

Thanksgiving morning Mom and I picked up Pop. She hadn't been to Mayberry before; I showed her around before we came back here. After we ate, we played several games of dominoes, with Pop and me partnered against Mom and John. Mom plays cut-throat. John plays for fun, but gloats when he wins. Pop likes to win, too, but gloats more with more subtle than John…well, not really.

I'm essentially the "dummy," because I don't keep track of what's been played, which means I often give away points, which means whoever partners with me, usually loses with me. And we got whupped bad. Pop thought about disowning me, but decided he'd have another piece of pecan pie instead.

Not long after the second belly-stuffing of the day, he wanted to go back to Mayberry. Either he was tired or he just wanted to unsnap his jeans—or both.

I know I was exhausted. Mom had gotten up several times during the night to use the bathroom, which disturbed my sleep. The sound of flushing in the main bathroom *roars* in the half-bath in our bedroom, sometimes making me sit straight up in bed.

Somewhere around 3 a.m., since I was awake anyway, I stuck the turkey in the oven to be sure it would be over-baked and dry six hours later. I got up a couple more times to baste it with a spoon, which wasn't easy, but I don't have a baking syringe-squirter.

However, I *can* tell you from past experience that basting with a spoon works better than trying to baste by rubbing a stick of butter over a turkey that's been in the oven for an hour, because the melting butter- stick will slip from your fingers and land on the oven floor, where it will sizzle and burn, fill the kitchen with smoke, and set off the smoke alarm—not just that time but for the next several times you use the oven.

I would baste with a fork before ever basting with a stick of butter again. "Dummy," yes; stupid, no.

Back to the present: John returned Pop to Mayberry, after which we dragged out the old Trivial Pursuit game. My fuzzy, sleep-deprived brain wasn't functioning real well. In fact, I was so pathetic that Mom and John started giving me two guesses plus hints—in between laughing at me. I started out way behind, but wound up beating both of them. Ha! Make fun of me, will they! (OK, OK, so I like to gloat, too.)

Late Friday morning the three of them drove to Tyler, but instead of staying overnight as planned, the men came back that evening. It had rained so much down there that the ground was too mushy for Pop to walk on safely.

Well, that was only part of it. Pop said he wanted to see Nancy Lee, then refused to go, which ticked off John. If he wasn't going to spend the afternoon with her, John saw no point in hanging around.

Sunday morning Pop called to report that Mildred, who was in the group picture Mary Ann took just last week, had died of a heart attack. "We're like family here," he said, "so everyone's pretty shook up."

This morning—it's Monday now—we saw Dr. A. While we were waiting in the exam room, I not only noticed Pop's hands looked dry and cracked, but how enormous they were. The tips of my fingers don't even reach his first knuckles. Big hands. Need to get him some lotion …that's my way of hedging into a confession.

As he went into the exam room ahead of me, I handed a note to the nurse and quietly asked her to have Dr. A read it before he came in. I'd written, "Please tell Pop he needs to walk more and cut down on snacks." He won't listen to John and me, but maybe he'd listen to Dr. A—who worked in the suggestions without snitching on me— maybe because Pop gained eleven pounds since his last visit. Wow! He's up a total of twenty-three pounds since May.

Might have something to do with the thirteen grams of fat and thirty-nine grams of carbs in each Little Debbie brownie. He's been eating at least four a day in addition to meals and other snacks.

Dr. A looked at a big, red, raised area on Pop's back. He squeezed it lightly to test it, said it was a sebaceous cyst that had gotten big enough to draw blood to the surface. He put on rubber gloves and squeezed a little harder, and—yuck.

"Sebaceous cyst," I said, "that's just a fancy word for a pimple, isn't it?"

"That's it," said the Cute One.

"I thought you weren't supposed to squeeze pimples," I challenged.

"I'm a doctor," he said, giving me a conspiratorial grin. "I know how to squeeze. We doctors can do anything we want to." Cute *and* a sense of humor!

"Ah-h-h, the truth finally comes out!"

He laughed. He gave Pop a flu shot, then sent him to the lab to siphon blood for more extensive calcium-level blood tests.

Moving on to this afternoon: Pop had those three cavities filled at Dr. B's, who also adjusted his temporary partial again. We were almost back to Mayberry before he told me it was still loose. I wouldn't turn around. He'll just have to rattle his teeth until we can go back again.

Thursday, November 30:

Sing along with Pop

Pop called yesterday. "Did you and John send me a birthday present?"

"No, why?"

"Somebody sent me a box of pens and some shredded money."

"Oh! Those must be from Sue, a lady I know. She told me she was going to send you a gift." (Sue is on my rubberstampers list.)

"Can I give some to the ladies?"

"Could you wait until tomorrow so I can see all of it first?"

"Oh, sure, Barbara."

Today Winona hosted her Sing Along in House 2. By the time I arrived, she had already started the show and was playing to a packed living room. I was pleased to see Pop already in the audience.

Some of the ladies shook maracas; they wore the fancy brimmed and flowered hats Winona provided. Pop waved a flag and shimmied a tambourine. Winona divided us into two teams to play "Name That Tune." The game was tied, three to three; tensions ran high. Then "Jingle Bell Rock" blared. No one recognized it except me, but I got close to Pop's ear and told him the name. He called it out, and our side won.

"Yea, Pop!" He grinned at me and mouthed, "Thank you."

Afterwards I walked one of the ladies back to House 4 because she was nervous about getting lost. I told her I sure understood because I tended to get lost, too. That alarmed her. She wanted to walk *me* back to House 2. I finally convinced her that I'd be fine, but I think she watched until she saw me reach the porch.

Inside, Pop was talking to Miss Bess. I didn't interrupt them, but went directly to his room. He had emptied the big mailing box from Sue onto his bed. I saw several decorated pens, large "matchbooks" containing pouches of shredded money, *and* four boxes of Little Debbie brownies. He had *not* mentioned the snacks on the phone yesterday.

When he walked into his room and saw the brownies, he muttered, "Dang! I meant to put those away." Made me laugh. You see, John and I started rationing Little Debbie because Pop won't ration himself. He can polish off three boxes in four days. No wonder his pants don't fit.

He sat in his chair; I covered him with all the goodies, and took pictures for us and Sue. Because it was only three days until his birthday, I relented and set aside one entire package for him to pig out on.

As I gathered up the rest to re-pack the mailing box, I thought, "Shouldn't there still be three boxes here?" I looked at the one I'd put on the bed's headboard, then looked over at Pop sitting innocently in his recliner. No boxes on his lap. Hmm-m...

I walked over and looked on the other side of his chair, and found the box he had surreptitiously slipped out of sight. He looked surprised.

"How did that get down there, Barbara?"

"As if you didn't know, you old rattlesnake."

He chuckled in the face of defeat. Should I have left it there? Probably. But I didn't. Sorry. One box to gorge on, but not two.

An almost-82 year-old man ought to be able to eat anything he wants, but I fear for his heart and arteries. Death by brownies may be the way Pop wants to go, but neither John nor I are ready to lose him.

Friday, December 1:

Lunch with Pop

I called him this morning to see if he wanted to run some errands with me.

"No," he allowed in his slow-talking drawl, sounding just a little vague. "I don't think I need anything."

"You could go just to get out."

"No-o-o-o-o, I think I'll just stay here and watch some TV. I'd just slow you down."

Well, sometimes I don't like to insist, so I told him I'd be over a little later with his December rent check. Just as well he didn't come with me. He would never have been able to climb into the tow truck: I came out of the drugstore to find my car wouldn't start. Click click zilch, then just zilch.

Of course I'd left my cell phone at home. The pay phone outside the store didn't work. I went inside where I saw the nice Dr. Pepper man restocking a vending machine, and begged him for a jump. He told me he was faithful to his wife, but he came outside with me anyway. I got the battery cables from my trunk, and he hooked them up.

The car still wouldn't start. I went back inside once more and begged the use of the store phone to call the Auto Club, then begged the use of their restroom. All that begging on those hard floors made my knees sore.

Gosh, the tow truck arrived in only fifteen minutes—probably a speed record. Hauled car and me across town, where the repair place found a loose battery cable. Fixed it up in a jiffy.

I finally made it to Mayberry, said "Hi!" all around, then took the empty chair next to Pop. Everyone was still eating lunch, and Gabriella, the house manager, asked if I'd like some. Sounded good— all that begging had worked up my appetite, too. She fixed me a plate.

Miss Frances sat to my left. She used to be a world traveler, and occasionally breaks into the Spanish she learned while living in South America. She's ninety-three now and has no short-term memory. She always asks if Pop is my father, and I tell her he's been my father-in-law for twenty-nine years, and he's more father to me than my dad is. Within a couple of minutes she repeats her question, and I just say, yes, he's my dad.

She asked me again today. This time when I told her he's my dad, she said, "Then how can you be so pretty when he's so ugly?" Everyone laughed. I think she actually set me up!

When Pop told me he was almost out of deodorant, I couldn't resist. "You had your chance to go with me and get some. You blew it. When you run out, you're just going to have to stink—unless...I know! Maybe Margaret could start giving you a bath every day instead of just Monday, Wednesday and Friday."

Margaret, who was sitting across from me, said she didn't come in Tuesday or Thursday. I suggested she give him a bath twice a day on the other three days. Pop had been quiet until then.

"I thought you were supposed to be on my side, Barbara," he said, as he r'ared back in his chair. "I don't want no bath twice a day, and I don't see why I can't go six weeks without one anyway. This every other day bathing is for ducks!"

Gabriella rescued him by serving dessert—bowls of vanilla ice cream topped with strawberry syrup. Pop received three scoops of ice cream, not one. Margaret protested, "Why should you get that much just because you're bigger?" She went to the side counter and cut a piece of leftover cake and brought it back to the table, gloating, "Ha, ha—I have ice cream *and* cake."

"That doesn't hurt my feelings," Pop snorted, "because I don't want cake anyway. And I still have more ice cream than you do."

Old folks may lose their memories, but their hearts remember how to be kids.

Sunday, December 3:

Pop's birthday

When I called him first thing this morning, he answered with, "Mr. Blanks' residence, Mr. Blanks speaking."

I started singing, "Happy Birthday Mr. Blanks, Happy Birthday Mr. Blanks," etc., then threw in "Happy Birthday, Pop!" at the end. He laughed and told me he hadn't recognized my voice until he heard me say "Pop." Yes, I sing that badly.

John picked him up right after lunch, and they drove around Garland for awhile. I didn't go with them because an out-of-town friend chose this weekend to be in town, and today was the only day we could get together. We played for four hours, then I had to get home for Pop's birthday dinner.

I was surprised to see he had his cane with him. He said he'd been walking more—just like he was supposed to—and felt strong enough to use it again. He still looked pretty unsteady to me, but his walker was back at Mayberry. Maybe if I walked behind him I could break his fall if he lost his balance? Didn't want to think about what I could break if he fell and landed on me.

He wanted to try a nearby chicken place that was open only in the evenings and on Sundays. Unfortunately, we discovered they closed early on Sunday—like two hours before we arrived. Because he had chicken on his mind, Pop couldn't decide between

91

Whataburger or Luby's, or some other place. I finally said I was hungry and getting cranky, which is when John decided we were going to Luby's. He's skeered of me when I'm hungry-cranky and rightly so. It's a low blood-sugar thing.

After eating, we drove around looking at Christmas lights. Not too many up yet, but Pop said he enjoyed himself.

He turned eighty-two today.

Monday, December 4:

After-birthday blues

Pop's birthday gloves were too small. I offered to take him to Walmart so he could return them and pick out another pair. When he grabbed his cane, I asked him to please use his walker instead, explaining if someone bumped into him or if he lost his balance, I wouldn't be able to stop him from falling. He acknowledged my concerns, and reluctantly set the cane aside.

He seemed fine until we were walking toward the store entrance, when he asked me, "Has it been fifteen years since Pat died?"

"No, Pop, just ten."

He stopped walking and started crying. He and Mother Pat had been married over forty years when she died unexpectedly a week after surgery on her broken collar bone. (She'd fallen down their porch stairs.) Partly he was missing her—and maybe partly because his girlfriend Nancy Lee is angry with him because he wouldn't see her at Thanksgiving. The holiday season is always more difficult after you've lost someone you love, and maybe he was feeling more alone than usual.

His breakdown lasted only a few seconds, and then he was ready to move forward again. In the face of everything that life has thrown at him, Pop has always moved ahead.

He tried on several pairs of gloves and finally settled on a pair he liked. We went back to Mayberry after that. He just didn't feel like going anywhere else.

Friday, December 8:

Short update

Dr. A reported that Pop's calcium level was still high, but not unacceptably so, and could even be normal for him.

Meanwhile, he's still walking and trying to lose some weight because he's not real happy about having his brownies rationed. He said he might have to be extra nice to "his" ladies in order to get some "sugar" that way. He grinned and glanced sideways at me to see if I was falling for it.

"Little Debbie's already given you a lot of sugar, Pop."

He licked his lips. "She sure was tasty, too."

If that man was as fast on his feet as he is with his mouth, I'd never be able to keep up with him!

Thursday, December 14:

Pop gets out after being iced in

Most of the Dallas area had been shut down for three dreary days due to one of our rare Texas ice storms, but today—today the sun took center stage and sang a Roger Miller tune that do-wacka-do'd us right between the eyes.

Roller skating in buffalo herds or on slippery sidewalks was definitely out, but the ice had melted off the roads enough to make driving safe, so I called Pop.

"Want to get out for awhile?"

"You bet!" He dropped the phone. I swear I heard him laying rubber with the wheels of his walker. He was waiting for me on the front porch. "What took you so long?" he asked.

"I put on shoes." He looked down, grimaced, and went back inside to change slippers for shoes.

First stop: the dentist. Pop's temporary partial was still loose. Dr. B discovered one of the wire "hooks" had broken off—undoubtedly from metal fatigue when that tech had tried to adjust it before. No way to repair it. Oh well, he can still eat. He'll be OK until he gets his permanent partial in January.

From there we went to browse the dollar store where Pop found those rubber snakes a few months ago. He needed birdseed, and I put several bags in the cart. As we were getting ready to check out, he thought an ice cream bar would really hit the spot. Sounded good to me, too.

No stack of tables to sit on like before, so we were going to eat in the car. But as we left the store, Pop saw an iron park bench in front of the restaurant next door. He suggested we sit there.

He walked over to the bench. I put the birdseed in the trunk, grabbed my gloves from the front seat, and joined Pop. Now mind you, it's December, the bench was in deep shade, and the wind was blowing briskly and steadily. The afternoon had gotten dismally cold.

But there we sat, shoulder-to-shoulder on a bottom-freezing iron bench, eating our ice cream bars, and enjoying every single bite.

Thursday, December 21:

Pop and the Christmas party

We caught part of the Sing Along with Winona before leaving to have Pop's hearing aids serviced. One didn't work because either he or John had put the battery in wrong and no one could get it out. Even the technician struggled before finally managing to remove it.

She cleaned the aid, put in a new battery, then looked in Pop's ears with a special light-camera that projected his ear wax in glorious color on the monitor screen. She didn't clean his ears—guess she just enjoyed the show.

Anyway, as he inserted the hearing aid, it split in half; some inside wires snapped. For something so expensive, it sure is fragile. Off for repair once again.

From there we ran some errands, one of which was stopping by my boss's house because I'm cat-sitting for her while she's out of town. Pop stayed in the car while I checked on the cats and took care of things inside. When we left, instead of going (the) right (way), I turned left—only to discover we couldn't go directly back to the main street.

After we meandered for awhile, Mr. Smart Alec asked, "Are we wandering around in circles again?"

"Hey!" I protested, smooth talker that I am.

Mayberry held their Open House Christmas Party tonight. When John and I arrived, all the ladies were gathered in the living room because some group had come a-caroling. Where was Pop? In his room watching TV.

I was rude and took his flipper away, turned off the TV, and told him to haul his rosy red behind outside and join the festivities. (I'm Bossy Barb, the elf Santa doesn't talk about.)

The owners of Mayberry Homes had holiday-decorated vases of flowers delivered to all four houses, one vase for each resident. Dianne also bought sweatshirts for everyone. Her color selections seemed perfect for each of the ladies and Pop. Dianne has a good heart. She could run Mayberry while keeping herself separate from the residents, but she knows them all by name, knows their histories, and she really cares about them.

Mary Ann delivered the framed cosmetic-party portraits yesterday. The families should be pleased with their presents. I wrapped up sachets for the ladies—token gifts, to be sure, but at least they had something extra under the tree.

Well, sad to say, John and I were the only family members who attended the House 2 party. I felt a little awkward at first. Some people (like Mary Ann) seem to have a knack for interacting with ten people at the same time. I don't. But I helped Dianne serve food, then after a couple of ladies went to their rooms, the rest gathered around one table where it was cozier and easier to talk.

We learned that Miss Frances used to be a golf pro—that's one reason she traveled so much—and a dance teacher. Miss Bess and her daughter were going to Memphis to spend Christmas with her son. Miss Lela couldn't remember how old she was, but Miss Helen, who's 83, told Lela she's 93. Lela and Bess almost got into a fight, because Lela tried to take Bess's sachet, thinking it was hers.

Frances kept trying to get Pop to kiss her—she's so funny. Dianne drew me aside to tell me that during the ice storm a few days ago, Bess suggested everyone should cuddle up in the same bed in order to keep warm. Frances said the only person with a bed big enough to hold all of them was Pop.

Pop deadpanned that at one time he could have handled nine women in one bed, but he wasn't sure he could now.

Sunday, December 24:

Two changes of plans

John, who had not had a real good day on Friday, took a nap after supper. An hour later he dragged himself, in his underwear, out to the living room to finish waking up; then he groaned and moaned as he went back to the bedroom to dress before going for a walk. I followed him.

"You look like you need a hug," I said, and threw my arms around him. I was pressed against his chest when—without missing a beat—he pulled a t-shirt over his head, then down over my head and upper body. He stooped to get his pants and proceeded to pull them on —all the while I was trapped under his shirt, laughing so hard I could barely breathe.

"I'm drooling on you," I said.

"Yuck!" He pulled up his t-shirt and released me. Silly man.

After his walk, John asked if it would bother me if we had Christmas at home. It just didn't make sense to him to load two cars with food, clothes and paraphernalia for three people and a dog, plus presents for five, just to spend two nights in Tyler.

He only voiced what I'd been thinking all along but didn't mention because usually he likes going to Tyler. I called my mom, who is amazingly adaptable, and asked if she'd come to us instead of us going to her. She had no problem with it—which meant that just like Thanksgiving—this would be the first time in twenty-nine years John and I would spend Christmas in our own home.

He and Pop went to Tyler yesterday, intending to spend the night because Pop planned to take Nancy Lee out for a catfish dinner that evening. They met Mark for lunch in the afternoon. Then, for unknown reasons, Pop decided not only didn't he want to take Nancy Lee to dinner, but didn't want to see her at all, even though he had a present for her.

Since he didn't want to do the girlfriend thing—again—John got annoyed with him and didn't want to stay the night—again. He called my mom. "Can you be ready to go in the next hour or so?"

"Oh, sure. I'm already mostly packed."

They arrived home just in time for supper, but Pop wanted to go back to Mayberry to eat. I think he thought John was a little peeved with him. He was right. So it was just us three for the meal, after which Mom and I played games while John exercised the TV flipper.

Then we all settled down for a long winter's sleep…

+++++

Mom and I went to church with John—one of my gifts to him because I don't attend. Truth is, I'm not a Christian, even though John and Pop are. I'm a failure at accepting the basic precepts of Christianity, without which you technically can't be a Christian. John calls me a pagan, but I'm not that either. I'm somewhere in-between.

Anyway, Pop didn't want to go with us, so we picked him up after the service. He and I partnered in dominoes. Our smart-aleck opponents scoffed at us because they were scoring twenty and thirty points at a time and figured they'd beat us easy—but we beat them both games by "nickel and dime-ing" our way up to five hundred points. Rub it in, rub it in!

Right now Mom is in the guest/junk room taking a nap. John (who actually washed the dishes after dinner) just went back to our bedroom for a nap. Charlie is sleeping by the front door. Pop is pushed back in the recliner watching an old western—with his eyes closed.

So what am I—who had trouble going to sleep, who woke up at 3:30 a.m., put the turkey in the oven way too early (do you detect a pattern here?), who woke again before six to let out the dog and check the turkey, who only dozed until 7:30 before getting up to walk Charlie, who went to church before having a chance to eat breakfast, then came home to put the meal together and get it on the card table, whose eyes are burning now from lack of sleep—so what am I doing?

Checking out the Rubberstampers List e-mails I didn't have a chance to look at yesterday. I should be taking a nap, too. Duh!

+++++

Later...

I finally succumbed and dozed off over the keyboard until the house started stirring again. John took Charlie for another walk. Mom staggered out of her room and parked on the couch. Pop woke up, struggled out of the recliner and went to the bathroom. When he returned, I asked if they wanted to go for a walk, too. Mom wouldn't budge out into the cold, but Pop was willing. I helped him bundle up, and as we headed out the door, I told him John was walking Charlie, so I was walking him.

"Is Charlie on a leash?" he asked.

"Yep."

"Well, maybe I should be on a leash, too."

97

"Yeah, you are a wild one, aren't you, Pop?" That tickled him.

After we walked uphill to the corner, I challenged him to a race. In a spurt of energy, he lifted his walker off the sidewalk and zoomed ahead of me. I had to hurry to catch up! We reached the end of the next block, crossed the street to go back the other way, and saw John and Charlie coming toward us. Charlie had tracked us from the house.

Pop stepped on the scales after his walk. He's at 205—and it shows. He said he weighs a hundred seventy-something naked, according to the scale at Mayberry. Uh-huh. Ain't no way his clothes weigh thirty pounds.

We opened our presents Christmas Eve. My sister sent Pop some snack cakes, and Mom gave him chocolate-covered cherries. He started "noodging" me—wondering if he was going to get to take his snacks back to Mayberry.

John and I are not playing Scrooge. We even put a whole box of Little Debbie brownies in his stocking for Christmas morning.

"Yes, Pop, you get to keep all your Christmas goodies," I said. "Maybe you can share some of them with the ladies at Mayberry."

"Not a chance!" he declared.

Monday, December 25:
Christmas Day with Mom—but mostly with Pop

It felt so strange to be spending our very first Christmas Day here at home that I'm going to tell you a story about a Christmas Past before telling you about our Christmas Present. (Ho! Ho! Ho!)

It was four years ago and our first one with Charlie. We were, of course, at Pop's in Tyler. That first night Charlie woke me up twice, whimpering from nightmares—probably being ganged up on by all the gophers whose holes he'd dug up during the day.

I got up to use the bathroom. Just as I dozed off again, the sound of something gnawing wood under the floor jarred me alert—undoubtedly a giant rat trying to gain entrance to the house. I finally relaxed enough to doze off again—and John snored right in my ear.

Charlie woke me way too early because isn't early the best time for a walk? Pop's yard wasn't fenced, and back then, Charlie wasn't yet trained enough to be trusted off-leash. He checked out all the bushes in front of the house before we wandered around back. Like the front porch, the back porch was built up high, with six steps at both ends, and protected by a generous cover. In addition, Pop had nailed a handy wooden shelf to the outside of the top railing.

It started sprinkling. I moved under the shelter of the overhang. The soft piles of dirt around the porch posts forced me to watch my footing, and—

Wham!

I cold-cocked myself. I dropped the leash and grabbed my head, trying to hold my brains in, trying not to die, positive that damn shelf had thrust itself all the way through my skull.

Unrestrained, Charlie wandered off in the direction of a wire-strand fence that bordered Pop's property. I'd forgotten it was there—and that it was electrified; low current, but—hey, wet ground plus wet dog equals great conductivity.

Wet nose sizzled. Charlie screamed, dancing in place, not knowing which way to go. I immediately forgot I was dying and called him. He ran to me in a zigzag crouch, still squealing. Together we wobbled to the porch steps and sat. I put my left arm protectively around him while I cradled my concussion with my right hand.

He licked anxiously at my face and snuffled. Eventually he stopped trembling; my brain stopped twirling. We walked around awhile longer, but he wouldn't go near the fence again. I opted not to walk under any more overhangs.

Now, back to this Christmas in Garland. Because the weather was supposed to deteriorate (freezing rain, sub-freezing temperatures), Mom wanted to go home fairly early. After opening stockings, playing two games of dominoes, and eating a lunch of leftovers, John and Mom took off for Tyler.

Pop thought he should "get out of your way" and go back to Mayberry, but I wouldn't let him. No way was he going to spend Christmas away from family, even though he mostly watched John Wayne movies and slept. I started putting the house back together, checking on him periodically to see if he wanted or needed anything.

We ate dinner-roll turkey sandwiches for an afternoon snack, then he ate two of his Little Debbie brownies in quick succession. I'm sure he feared I'd take them away. I hate being the villain. (By the way, it didn't feel right to dole out his treats, so John and I have been giving Pop one box of brownies every Sunday. Now it's his choice as to how long it lasts.)

John got home around five. I fixed regular turkey sandwiches for supper—which is exactly what he had his mouth set for. After we ate, Pop was ready to go back to Mayberry, but first he and John drove around in the rain and looked at Christmas lights.

John was so butt-sprung from five hours of driving that when Charlie wanted to go for his nightly walk in the cold and continuing rain, they went.

Right after they left, Steve, an old Air Force buddy of John's called. Steve had driven down from Kansas a couple of years ago and stayed with us for a week. He's a wellspring of funny stories. After we talked for awhile, he told me to tell John that while he was out walking the dog, we'd had a brief but torrid affair.

That's exactly what I did. John called Steve back. I heard him laughing at one point and saying, "Yeah, she told me that as soon as I walked in the door."

Hope your Christmas Day was as fun, as warm and cozy, as funny, and as nice as ours was.

Friday, December 29:

Pop is sick

Pop felt poorly Tuesday evening. He felt even worse after he turned on his side to put his book down and fell out of bed. Dianne heard the WHUMP! She hurried to his room and helped him up.

Wednesday morning she called to say he'd sweated through his clothes trying to get out of his recliner, and called again later to report he'd "fallen all over his room." John saw him that evening. Pop coughed a little, but didn't say he felt bad.

I went over Thursday to take him out for a haircut. He was hanging onto his door frame, trying to find his hearing aid, which was already in his ear. When he let go of the frame to turn around, he swayed and tilted backwards. He'd have fallen if I hadn't steadied him.

"Let's forget the haircut, Pop. I don't think you can make it to the car." He didn't argue. He staggered over to his chair and sat. He said if he just rested awhile, he'd be OK.

Around suppertime Dianne called yet again; she thought he had the flu. I phoned Dr. A's office, and they worked Pop in as the last patient of the day. He could barely walk by then. John helped him into Mother Pat's old wheelchair—we've been storing it in his closet. That sure simplified getting him out to the truck and into the clinic.

Not only was his temperature a hundred-two, but his head and lungs were congested. When Dr. A said it could be the flu, I put my hands on my hips and allowed, "It better *not* be. You gave him a flu shot last month."

"You're right about that," he said, grinning while he swabbed Pop's throat. He looked at his watch. "The culture takes twenty minutes, but the lab closes in ten." He laughed. "They're not going to be happy with me—but they'll get over it." And he took the culture to the lab himself.

John, who had not seen Dr. A before, said he wasn't nearly as cute as he'd been led to believe by the Mayberry ladies and by me. He just has no appreciation of the finer views of life.

+++++

Dianne called this morning, sounding stressed—Pop was dizzy and disoriented, and so weak it took two people to get him sitting up and out of bed so he could use the bathroom. She thought he should be in the hospital—and why hadn't Dr. A given him a shot?

"A shot for what?" I asked. "He doesn't have an infection." I called the doc's office again to ask about Pop's new symptoms. Dr. Angel Face called back in short order. He said dehydration can cause dizziness and confusion. A-ha!

When I got to Mayberry, Pop was lying in bed. After I made him drink most of a glass of water, he was able to get up and totter into the bathroom by himself.

He admitted he hadn't been drinking much of anything because he was tired of going to the bathroom so often. Oh, great! No liquids and a fever. No wonder he was dehydrated, dizzy and disoriented.

Pop hadn't wanted breakfast, but thought he "could eat a little something" when lunch time rolled around. Since we didn't know if he was contagious, he ate in his room. He sat on the edge of his bed; I sat next to him, my right arm around him trying to support his back, while I steadied his plate with my left hand. He slumped into my shoulder. I had to brace my feet to keep us from falling over sideways.

He really was hungry. He ate everything on his plate and wanted his dessert. He'll live.

101

Kellie, who had recently taken over as House Mother after Gabriella decided to step down, fixed a plate for me, too. Since it was cold by the time I got to it, I ate my dessert first—ice cream with peach cobbler. Didn't want it to get warm.

John and I swapped places after supper. He had a root canal this morning, and now he's spending the night in a recliner, just in case his dad needs him. Does he know how to have fun or what?

By the way, the throat culture results indicate it's not the flu. Something is going around that mimics it, but no one seems to know what it is. John and I have been popping echinacea and washing our hands like crazy, hoping that whatever Pop has will end with him. I don't have time to be sick, and I sure don't want to have to take care of John.

Actually, John is easy when he feels bad—he mostly sleeps. It's when he starts feeling better that he needs to be strangled.

Saturday, December 30:

Doing better

Neither man slept well last night because Pop got up at least eight times to use the bathroom. Today his temperature is close to normal, but his cough sounds liquid and he wheezes when he breathes. Still, he ate breakfast while sitting on the edge of the bed—without support. He even joked around a little.

He'd said his back ached, so I brought along a tube of pain-relief gel when I traded places with John after lunch. Courtney applied it—Pop enjoyed that. She's on duty over the entire weekend, and he likes her.

He walked around the circular hall a couple of times to get his blood pumping—just enough so he could take a nap. I tried to stay in the room with him and read a *RubberStampMadness* while he slept, but I'm not used to sitting still during the day. I finally wandered into the kitchen and helped Cortney clean up the lunch mess. I helped her serve supper and clean up afterwards, too.

John is staying the night with Pop again—just in case. He's so tired he might actually sleep. What a way to spend New Year's Eve.

Monday, January 1:

Happy New Year, y'all!

Usually I'm asleep before the New Year comes in, old fogey that I am, but I stayed up last night in case neighborhood celebratory noises gave Charlie the shakes, which they've done in the past.

Dead silence outside at midnight. I went to bed and drifted off. Someone set off some firecrackers—too drunk to know the time? Jarred me awake. I dozed again. Fifteen minutes later, more firecrackers exploded. Charlie couldn't handle it and came to my side of the bed. I let him jump up—hey, John wasn't there. Feeling comforted, he settled down immediately, so I had a warm body to snuggle up to after all.

Pop is starting the New Year off right—he's feeling much better. He actually got dressed and ate at the dining table this morning.

Hope y'all out there are feeling perky and able to sit up and take nourishment, too. If not, I'll try not to make too much noise while you're recovering from last night's festivities.

Tuesday, January 16:

A rant of this, a little of Pop

I had a mammogram appointment at the Women's Center yesterday. An hour-and-a-half after I signed in, I walked up to the counter and reminded the clerk, "You told me it would be just a few minutes. I arrived at the scheduled time. I upheld my end of the appointment contract. Why aren't you upholding yours?" She called someone in the back, then unconcernedly told me it would be another twenty minutes.

Something in her attitude made fury rise in me so fast I thought sure I had transformed into the Incredible Hulk. (Hmm-m-m, he looks green, but does he see red?) *Barely* maintaining enough control to not maim her, I pointed to the hall door and said, "I'm going out there for awhile," and left.

I walked off enough of my anger to be able to return and tell the girl I wanted to speak to whoever was in charge. She called to the back again, and a supervisor appeared a couple of minutes later. After hearing me out (and it was hard talking with my lips clenched around my control), she apologized, then said they'd had three emergencies and were running behind. Uh-huh. I didn't care.

"Then I should have been told that when I first checked in. I would have understood, but I was told it would just be a few minutes." She agreed with me, but it didn't mollify me. Maybe I doubted her sincerity?

Did I still want to get my mammogram today? Well, duh! After waiting for almost two hours I wasn't about to leave without one. The supervisor told me they were ready for me. She handled it … them ... herself. Let me tell you, never annoy the person who is about to squash the living jehosaphats out of your breasts. Maybe she didn't squeeze me any harder than the time a horse stepped on my foot and stayed awhile, but I wouldn't swear to it.

Guess what I saw after I left the x-ray room. All those way-behind-techs sitting around their work station, laughing, shooting the breeze and definitely not prepping anyone else.

Emergencies my boobies! Medical abuse is what it is. That's my rant and I'm sticking to it!

As for Pop, his lungs have cleared up. It's been raining all day, and since he couldn't get outside, he'd been feeling a little dark and dreary himself before Charlie and I went to see him this afternoon.

He enjoyed hearing about Charlie treeing a squirrel in our yard —and getting rain-drenched in the process. He wanted to know if we could go to Walmart so he could pick out a card for John's upcoming birthday. Most importantly, he was out of brownies.

Just a little visit, nothing special, except he was glad to see us, and we were glad to see him.

Friday, January 26:

Pop goes for Mexican

Pop was stuck at Mayberry all week because I had to work. I called him this afternoon and said, "It's party time! I'll pick you up on my way home." Handsome fella was ready and waiting for me on the porch.

He was also quick to tell me his brownie stash needed replenishing again, and wanted to know if he'd lost any weight yet. Our bathroom scales showed he'd lost five pounds. He thought he deserved at least two boxes of brownies a week now, but I suggested maybe he needed to lose another five pounds first. He was disappointed, of course, but didn't argue with me.

While Pop was still living in Tyler, he used to fix a microwave sausage and biscuit for breakfast, ate lunch at the Senior Center or picked up a burger somewhere, then ate brownies all evening. He didn't gain weight on that weird diet, and I don't think he connects three good meals plus snacks plus brownies with all his extra poundage.

We met John at the little Mexican restaurant Pop likes. As soon as he saw his son, he announced, "Since I've lost five pounds, Barbara told me I could have three or four boxes of brownies in my room now." My jaw dropped.

"You liar!" I sputtered.

"You mean you didn't tell me that, Barbara?" Mr. Innocence could barely contain his laughter.

"You know I didn't, you liar!" I said, trying to keep a straight face. Pop laughed, hugely enjoying his joke.

Later, toward the end of the meal, I watched as he used a teaspoon to scoop his salsa dip over the small portion of beans and tamale he had left. As he put the spoon down, I said, "You'd better put some of that on your rice, too."

He paused, looked up at me and grinned. "You think so?"

"Oh, yeah." He spooned on the rest of the sauce. He also bought a monstrous pecan praline at the register, and no, I didn't say a word.

John wanted to gas up the truck, so Pop drove back to Mayberry with me. That's when we had one of our more deliciously flavorful, high-class conversations.

me: What have you been up to all week, Pop?

Pop: Oh, mostly just eatin' and sleepin'.

me, deadpan: Yep, eatin', sleepin', and fartin'.

Pop, flabbergasted: *What* did you say?

me, laughing: Just eatin', sleepin', and fartin'.

Pop, disbelieving: That's what I thought you said!

Pop, pondering: You know, Barbara, I usually try to wait till I'm sitting on the commode before I fart now. Sometimes they come out "juicier" than I expect.

me, grinning: It's hard walking away and pretending someone else farted when they're juicy, isn't it?

Pop, laughing: Yep, it sure is.

Thursday, February 15:

Pop and the chauffeur

John and Mark both have birthdays in February. They let Pop buy their lunch in Longview last Saturday to celebrate. Other than that, he hadn't gotten out much recently because I've worked every day for the last three weeks.

So, today, in spite of all the rain, I picked him up about ten, intending to put an end to his long captivity.

First stop was Dr. A's office—lab only. It was past time for his calcium level to be rechecked. If it hasn't changed, we can figure "high" is normal for him.

Second stop was Dr. R's office to pick up a claim form they'd filled out for the cyst removal surgery. I've sent the claim in twice already, but Medicare refused to pay on the first submission, referencing anesthesia for eye surgery. Hello? What eye surgery? Eye teeth maybe? I resubmitted; they refused it again, saying the provider had to fill out the claim form. Why didn't they tell me that from the get-go?

Shaggy Man needed a haircut. He liked the last barber John took him to, and I can understand why. We could barely understand him because of his strong accent, but he treated Pop with respect. And unlike all the other barbers, he even trimmed the flyaway hairs in Pop's eyebrows and the little hairs sticking up along the edges of his ears.

After he was buffed and polished, and we were back in the car, I said, "OK, pretend you're rich." He snorted. "Now pretend I'm your chauffeur. I'll wear a cap if you want me to, but I draw the line at short skirts and low-cut blouses." His face tinged with red. "Your wish is my command, Sir. Where to?"

He said he needed birdseed. Since rain was pelting down, he opted to stay in the car while I dashed into the dollar store and bought twelve bags. The nice cashier not only went to the backroom to get some boxes to pack them in, but carried two of them out to the car for me.

Then Pop asked if there were any bookstores nearby. That's something you don't hear him ask very often—like never. He reads a few westerns and the newspaper, but that's about it. But he'd finished his three Louis L'Amour books and wanted more.

We drove to a nearby bookstore, where he picked out three he didn't think he'd read, but since he couldn't remember them, it really didn't matter.

Pop's growling stomach led us to Whataburger. "This is why your son loves me," I told him as he paid for my lunch. "I'm a cheap date."

After we ate, we made one more quick stop to pick his prescription refill. Well, not as quick as it would have been if the store hadn't moved its display of Little Debbie products. Had to find those—by special request—before we could check out. After that we headed back to Mayberry.

When Margaret learned we'd had lunch but no dessert, she offered us ice cream sandwiches. We each took one, then Kellie joined us at the dining table while we talked and ate.

I had to run after that. The Chauffeur was off-duty, but well-compensated for her time.

Friday, February 16:

Nothing but the tooth—

Pop tried out the toothless metal frame of his new permanent lower partial-plate today. Dr. B said it's easier to see how the piece fits that way—and it has to fit perfectly because it can't be changed once the teeth are set in.

After adjusting the frame, he cast an impression of Pop's upper gum line, then disappeared into his lab to shape wax over it. When he came back, he used a tiny "blowtorch" to soften the wax upper denture, inserted it into Pop's mouth, then had him close his jaw at precise intervals until finally his lower teeth pressed against the wax. He said it was easier to get a good fit and an accurate bite if both upper and lower dentures were made together like that.

When Dr. B, who should have been a sculptor, was satisfied with his handiwork, we picked out a tooth color that closely matched the few real teeth Pop has left. His new dentures will look way more natural than his old ones do.

"Wooo—eee, Pop!" I said. "When you get your new teeth, you're going to look *so* good that all the ladies at Mayberry are going to smooch on you."

He preened. "They already do."

Saturday, February 24:
Giving Mayberry the slip

Pop woke up late last night, urgently needing to use the toilet. As he hurried into his bathroom, he slipped on its vinyl floor—probably because he was only wearing socks—well, socks and underwear, but he wasn't walking on his underwear. He landed on his back.

His yell brought Dianne running to his room. She helped him up, and since he seemed to be all right, no one called us until this morning when he had trouble moving. Fortunately, because it was storming, we weren't already two hours along the road to Tyler to see my mom.

John took his dad to a Saturday urgent-care clinic, where they took two x-rays of his back, saw nothing damaged, gave him a pain shot, and sent him on his way.

He's sore and has a massive bruise along his entire back, but is otherwise OK. I took some pain relief gel over a little while ago. He won't mind having young Cortney rub it in.

Tuesday, March 13:
Poor pitiful me

I wasn't sure I'd live through Friday. My throat was a mess and I felt like warmed-over calf slobber. My throat looked like warmed-over calf slobber, too. I called my doctor's office.

"Hello, I'm dying. I need to see Dr McM." They could work me in at 1 p.m. Great. If I went in earlier and collapsed in the waiting room, I wondered if they would shove me out of sight until then.

Once there, I still had to wait close to an hour, but I was almost unconscious for most of it. The nurse came into the exam room, stuck a long swab down my throat—which made me cough in her face—and took a strep culture. Then the doctor came in.

"So you have a sore throat?" Dr. McM asked.

"No, this goes beyond 'sore.' We're talking real pain here."

She thought that was amusing. She looked at my throat.

"You have an ugly exudation," she said—only because in medical school they teach you not to say, "Gross! The dingle-dangle at the back of your throat is Slime City."

108

"Yeah, I know," I said—like it was something to be proud of.

It actually *was* strep. Dr. McM said a penicillin shot would leave me contagious for another 24 hours, but I'd feel better sooner than if I took pills. I opted for the shot. She tossed, "I'll let my nurse do the dirty work," at me as she left the room. She wasn't kidding.

Nurse had me lie face down on the table with my bare backside staring at the ceiling. She used a needle long enough to reach clear through to the front of my thigh, and pumped in the antibiotic—too much medicine to do a clean poke and squirt. All the while she told me about possible allergic reactions which could kill me (like I cared right then), so I should go back to the waiting room and sit on my sore hiney for at least twenty minutes before going home—just in case.

"Can't I just lie here and die?" I pleaded.

"Nope, pull up your pants and get out of here."

Well, I do feel a whole lot better now. I've been watching the recovery process with fascination. All the foam at the back of my throat wasn't spit—it was bacterial excretion. When it disappeared, I could see a patch of white over my left tonsil big enough to ski down.

This morning the snow is "melting" and patchy. I don't feel good, but don't feel sick either. Still better not get too close to Pop yet.

Monday, March 19:

Pop's in trouble

He got caught urinating into the bushes off the front porch. He was alone out there and thought no one could see him. Not good.

This came on the heels of a similar incident the last time he and John were in Tyler. They had stopped at the post office to check Pop's postal box for any unforwarded mail. John went inside. When he came back out, he saw his dad relieving himself on the front tire of the truck.

Pop's a country boy. He's used to whipping it out in the great outdoors. He had to go, knew he couldn't hold it long enough to reach a restroom, and well...John was not amused. He told his dad in no uncertain terms that he'd better not ever do that again because he could be jailed for indecent exposure.

When Dianne called about today's watering, John, who is normally pretty easy going, erupted—which he can actually do without raising his voice, although he does look like a rabid gorilla.

He confronted his dad, who only made John angrier by trying to make excuses for himself. Aside from reminding Pop that he could be arrested and/or thrown out of Mayberry, John pointed out that any of the ladies could have looked out a window—or walked out the front door—and seen him; Barbara—or someone else—could have pulled up in front of the house while he was "occupied." How embarrassing would *that* be? John warned him against ever pulling a stunt like that again.

I'm guessing Pop won't remember the reasons for not doing what he considers natural, but hopefully he'll keep it zipped up from now on.

By the way, I know I quite often bring up Pop's bladder, but you need to understand it's a major focus of his life. If we live long enough, we all travel full circle—from having no bladder control when we come into this world to losing bladder control as we head out the other way. It's a slippery slope we tread in this life—uphill, downhill and over the hill.

Wednesday, March 21:

Pop's choppers

Today was THE DAY. Pop got his new dentures.

A couple of weeks ago, when he told his brother about his new teeth, Mark congratulated him, then teased, "Hey, Johnny, why don't you give me those old things so I can use them."

Pop decided it would be a great joke to wrap them and give them to Mark as a gift.

I explained this to the tech when I asked her to clean the old teeth. I don't think she appreciated the humor, but Pop sat in that dental chair and grinned within an inch of his life, anticipating Mark's reaction.

Out with the old teeth, in with the new.

Dr. B set about fine-tuning the fit, sanding down the high spots, testing the bite, etc. He warned that a little more adjusting would be necessary as the teeth settled in, then left his assistant to show Pop how to insert and remove the lower partial.

110

To remove it, all he had to do was place his left thumb under the wire clasp and press up. When the left side released, the right would automatically pop off. To "install" it, he had to use both index fingers to press and click it into place.

He practiced the technique four times—which wasn't enough because he had trouble fingering the clasp, but I could tell the assistant wanted to get him out of the chair. I would have ignored her attitude if Pop himself hadn't been getting aggravated and frustrated with the whole procedure. He looked like he needed a break.

We left, and arrived back at Mayberry just as lunch was being served. I dropped him off, went to Walmart to pick up some items he needed, then returned to cut his hair for the first time. How did his Chauffeur become his Barber?

Well, over twenty years ago, when John still had hair and wore it longer, we bought a hair clipper kit so we could save money by having me cut his hair. I'd been doing a class job—considering I had never cut hair before—until the description of the function of the second attachment misled me into thinking it would cut only a little off the hair tips to even up the length. It didn't.

John got real still when I muttered, "Uh-oh." He didn't think it was nearly as funny as I did, nor as funny as the barber did, who laughed at the bare swath cut up the back of John's head. He said a lot of his business came from husbands whose wives tried to cut their hair.

John, however, has far less hair now than he did then, and he keeps what's left real short. Still, when he came home last week with a barber kit, I was surprised—but took the razor to his head with great aplomb. He looks magnificent. He showed off his haircut to Pop and asked if he'd mind if I cut his hair, too.

Pop, brave man, said he'd give me a shot—and if I botched it, he'd have me shot. Well, he and John have the Blanks' hairline: mostly bald. It's not like I can mess it up *too* badly.

Since Pop was sitting on the porch at Mayberry, and an outdoor electrical outlet was near the front door, I just plugged the razor in there. I shifted his chair, effectively blocking the entrance, but since I was now an experienced faux-barber, it didn't take long to shear the lamb. I even trimmed his eyebrows. He thought the price of the hair cut was just right…until I told him how much I expected him to tip.

Afterwards, I asked if he'd do a partial-plate removal demo for me—just to see if he could do it. He was agreeable, but first he wanted to practice eating again with his new teeth. A man needs to fortify himself before a challenge.

We scrounged up and devoured some leftover dessert—angel food cake rolled up with cherry pie filling—before going to his bathroom where he could stand in front of the mirror and see what he was doing.

The man struggled and struggled and struggled trying to get that partial out. He put too many fingers in his mouth; he tried to lift in the wrong places; he tried to lift the wrong side with the wrong hand. He took his new upper plate out so he'd have more room to maneuver—and almost dropped it.

He was getting mad. I suggested he stop for a minute and relax; he waited only a few seconds before he returned to the fray.

He finally got it unhooked and out. Man, *I* was sweating by then! "OK, put it back in."

He turned it this way and that, then tried to put it in upside down.

"The teeth point upwards, Pop." He snorted in disgust, flipped them over, and managed to click them in place.

"Good! Now take them out again." He gave me an exasperated look, which made me laugh, which made him grin. He took up the gauntlet again.

He struggled and he drooled and he struggled, but he got it out a little more easily. Back in again. He initiated the battle himself that time. Came out a little faster.

The clasp will gradually loosen, and he'll eventually get used to the procedure. John's over there now delivering bird seed. I hope he remembers to ask for a demonstration of Pop popping his new teeth.

His smile is different now.

Monday, April 9:

Surprises and challenges

I've mentioned Miss Obed, my boss's aunt, before—she's the lady Charlie and I would sometimes visit in House 3. Today Mona told me she died a week ago—just sort of tossed the news at me when I was doing some work in her office. I knew she hadn't been doing

112

well, but the news surprised me; got me all teary-eyed. She was a sweet lady.

+++++

Pop was anxious to deliver The Gift, which I had wrapped and ribboned for him. He and John got together with Mark in Tyler on Saturday. They had lunch at a Mexican restaurant where they've eaten before, but Pop keeps forgetting how sizzling the salsa is. According to John, he scooped a huge helping of it onto his tortilla chip and took a bite. Seconds later he started sweating; his face turned red.

"Wonder when they're gonna bring us something to drink," he said, trying to sound casual. He didn't fool John or Mark for a second. They turned red from laughing at him.

After Pop cooled off, he presented his brother with the gift of used teeth. Mark, apparently, was actually pleased to receive them— no surprised exclamations.

Seemed a little anti-climatic to me, but when I asked Pop about it this afternoon, his smile almost broke his cheeks. Whether Mark got the joke or not, Pop majorly relished it.

He also felt pretty pleased with himself because he likes the challenge of trying to talk "that old woman" out of his bath, and today he won. Margaret doesn't take any guff, and Pop likes to dish it out, so they go at it all the time. It's funny to hear how they fuss at each other, but one day he confided to me that he likes her.

I noticed his hearing aids were sticking out, which meant he put them in the wrong ears. I brought it to his attention. He swore he'd put them in right, but when he took them out and switched ears, he sheepishly admitted that not only did they feel better, but he could hear better, too.

I asked him if there was anything he wanted to do, or anywhere he wanted to go. He couldn't think of anything. And then he said that he didn't think he could ever live at home again. It's the first time he's acknowledged it. He said, "I have trouble climbing the porch stairs, and since I can't drive anymore—well, it just wouldn't be the same."

"Can you think of anyone who would be willing to be a paid companion and live with you at home?" He said no, that he was happy at Mayberry. Everyone was good to him—even "that old woman," meaning Margaret. He was content to stay where he was.

113

The best part was being near us; he really liked that. He talked about the last time he and John drove around for a couple of hours, which he enjoys more than when he drove around by himself.

Long before his car wreck Pop started having trouble dealing with ordinary household problems. If something didn't work properly or if anything interfered with his routine, it would throw him into a panic. He sometimes paid his bills late. I once found his unmailed income tax return in a pile of papers three months after it was due, even though I had done everything except actually mail it for him. He had also started calling us every night after someone he knew died but wasn't found for almost a week. He didn't want that happening to him.

He'd been trying to hand the responsibilities of home over to us for awhile, so I think he's relieved that we've finally accepted them.

Just before I left, he told me he still had a couple of brownies left from a week ago Sunday. That surprised me.

"I guess I could take them home with me," I said. He snapped his recliner upright.

"Oh, you wouldn't want to do that!"

"Gotcha, Pop."

"Doggone you, Barbara, you could stop an old man's heart talking that way."

Pop might be winding down, but Little Debbie can still crank him back up.

I laughed, kissed his bald head, and headed for the door. "I love you, Pop. See you later."

"Love you, too, Barbara."

Friday, April 20:

Pop walks through Kohl's

When I called on Wednesday, I dialed the house phone because it was lunchtime and knew Pop wouldn't be in his room. Kellie, chief cook and pamperer-of-residents, answered. I asked her to ask him if he'd like to get out for awhile this afternoon.

I could hear her talking to him, then saying, "It'd be good for you," meaning he was refusing my invitation since he always thinks he's too much trouble. When she came back on the line, I told her to tell him I'd whip his hiney if he didn't come with me. She relayed the message. Pop's afraid of me—ha ha. He decided to come after all.

About forty-five minutes later we hit the road. He'd never been to Kohl's Department Store, and while that's not the most exciting of destinations, I had three pairs of shoes I needed to return, and he was my captive, so we went. As we pulled into a parking space, he said,

"I don't want to slow you down, Barbara. I'll just wait for you in the car."

"Nuh-uh!" I told him. "Ain't no way you're staying in the car." I am *so* bossy. "Besides, you might see something you can't live without." He came in with me.

Of course I parked at the wrong entrance. He got his exercise and the Grand Tour as we slowly made our way to Customer Service, which was clear on the other side of the store.

He stopped every once in awhile to look at something that caught his eye. We were in the Men's section when I pointed out a display of patterned, silky boxer shorts.

"Hey, Pop, you should get some of these! Wooo-eee! You could give Margaret a thrill when you strip for your bath."

"She already gets a thrill when she sees me naked," Mr. Modest declared.

After we reached Customer Service, he rolled into the restroom; I returned the shoes. Finished with our business, we decided to complete the circuit of the store. As we headed around the other way, I heard the distinctive sound of Peggy Lynne, my wonderful friend-since-forever, calling my name.

Peggy Lynne is uniquely exuberant. A few years ago, after I dyed my hair for the first time, I came up behind her at Target and deliberately bumped her basket. She whirled around, saw me, and screamed, "You have red hair!"

"Yes, I know," I laughed, not at all surprised or embarrassed by her outburst. "Thank you for telling everybody in the store about it."

P.L. was on her way to Customer Service. Pop had met her a long time ago, and I think he actually vaguely remembered her. She *is* hard to forget. She told him how handsome he was, and how much his son looks like him. Pop blushed but ate it all up. We talked for a few minutes more then moved on.

Because of the narrow aisle, I was a little ahead of him when we approached a display of musical flower pots. I pushed a button on one as I went by. The flowers started bobbing and twirling. Pop and his walker stopped dead in their tracks. He'd not seen anything like them before.

As soon as that pot stopped playing, I pressed the button on one labeled "In the Mood." I did a little dance number for him. He grinned and clapped. Nothing like a floor show in the middle of Kohl's.

Back at the car, I asked him if there was anywhere he'd like to go so he wouldn't have to go back to Mayberry right away.

"Would it be too much trouble to go by my old house?" he asked. Of course not.

When John was thirteen, Pop couldn't find work in Tyler, but Texas Instruments in Dallas was hiring. He made the long commute for several months before he and Mother Pat bought a house in Garland. They lived there for twenty-eight years, but hung onto the family property (about fifteen acres just south of Tyler), land that Pop's grandfather bought in the 1800s, right after the Civil War. Then, a couple of years after Pop retired, he and Mother Pat sold the Garland house and moved back to their land.

After she died, I stayed with Pop for awhile to help him get things sorted out. John would have stayed, too, but he had to go back to work.

After that, whenever we went to Tyler, naturally I'd spend most of my time with my mom. Pop and I probably talked more on the phone than we did in person—until his car wreck.

Anyway, we left Kohl's and drove to his old neighborhood of small wood-frame houses. They've all been renovated in recent years as new families moved in. His old house and garage have siding now, and a picture window has replaced the garage door. Could be it's been converted to a workshop or apartment. What he saw made Pop feel good.

He pointed out houses and named the people who used to live there and told me a little about them. He can't remember Miss Margaret's name, but he remembers his old neighbors. After that he was ready to go back to Mayberry, his new neighborhood.

+++++

It's Friday already. I went over this glorious spring afternoon to cut Pop's hair again. He hasn't fired me yet, so he must like the way it looks. Probably he likes not having to struggle into a barber chair, too.

We sat and talked for awhile afterwards, then I had to get home, where I washed the car, washed the dog, washed the dog-towels and bathroom rug, then washed my hair.

Margaret had helped Pop bathe this morning. He wasn't wearing fancy boxer shorts from Kohl's, but I still thought I heard a "Wooo-eee!" blowing in the wind.

Sunday, April 29:
Sing along with Pop and the bouncing birthday girl

Pop fooled me. I didn't have to shake him out of his chair so we could attend the Sing Along with Winona. He pulled open his door just as I knocked, startling both of us. He was ready to go.

Winona always wears a dress, heels, and one of her old-fashioned Easter-bonnet brimmed hats. She obviously loves these old folks: she holds their hands and "dances" with them; she hugs gently; she asks questions about what it was like "back then."

This time she brought birthday booklets that listed news items from past years. Three ladies had birthdays in April—as did I. We each called out our birth years, and Winona read selected items from those years. One study showed that women were safer drivers than men. The women cheered, but Pop jeered.

"Boo-o-o-o!"

I didn't know the man was a fool! "Pop! You're outnumbered!"

If those women could have gotten out of their seats and through the maze of walkers and wheelchairs, he'd have been dead meat. He just grinned, mightily pleased with the uproar he'd caused. He reminded me of Charlie—who will stand on one side of a fence while some dog barks in his face, getting all riled, then he'll whirl away and trot off, sporting a huge grin. Like puppy, like Grampy.

When I got home after the Pop-roast, there was a message on the machine from my calls-me-if-she-needs-me boss, Mona. Could I work Friday? Awww, man! I didn't want to work on my birthday.

I almost said no, but then realized I'd be doing laundry and cleaning toilets if I stayed home. Work suddenly sounded like a good idea. I decided to go in. I figured no one knew it was my birthday, so I wasn't expecting any special treatment.

But Friday morning, all the designers except Allison presented me with cards, a pot of miniature roses, and a box of glazed donuts—those surprised me because everyone out there had been trying to eat healthier for the last several months.

Every time I've gone in I've "complained" about the dearth of the previously plentiful chocolate. The last time I worked, though, Allison anticipated my "whine" and brought me a snack-bag of M&M's. I polished them off, then put the empty packet on her desk along with a note asking if it was refillable. Later, when she returned to her office and found it, I could hear her laughing.

So, Allison didn't give me a birthday card. She gave me a gift bag filled with an assortment of snack-size candy bars. My cheeks hurt from smiling.

After the party Mona worked me hard. I carried heavy file boxes into a hot little storage room, helped move five 4-drawer, jam-packed file cabinets, and carted discontinued granite samples out to the trash bin. Good thing I got to sit down and do paperwork all afternoon because I could barely stand upright after all that. I was still dragging when I left for the day.

Got home to find singing birthday messages from my mom and friend Peggy Lynne—and a message from a woman at Medicare I've been trying to talk with for two weeks—RATS! Called my friend Sandy in Oklahoma, who had actually left a message yesterday but I hadn't had a chance to call her back.

And I returned my best friend Nan's call. When Nan started singing Happy Birthday, I joined in. Neither one of us can carry a tune worth a flip, but we have a great time un-harmonizing together.

By that time John was home. I don't believe in cooking on my birthday—or anyone else's if I can avoid it. I'd asked Pop a couple of days ago if he wanted to eat out on my birthday.

"Sure!" he said.

"That's good," I told him, "because you're buying."

"Oh, I am, am I?" He laughed.

"Yep—it's your birthday present to me."

After John got home, I called Pop to see if he was ready to go to supper. He didn't sound real good. He said he thought he might be getting a cold, and wasn't very hungry.

"Would you rather not go?"

"No, no, might be good for me to get out."

We picked him up and drove to a cafeteria—hey, as long as I don't have to cook, I don't care where we eat. Pop didn't think he wanted much, but he still selected a big tossed salad, cornbread, chicken-fried steak, veggies, and a slice of apple pie.

A server carried his tray, followed John to a booth, and set it down. John, who was still hyped from work, unloaded his own tray and started eating before Pop and I caught up.

He used his walker and the table's edge to support himself as he sat on the bench seat. I moved his dishes out of arm's way (i.e. kept his elbow out of his food), and slid in next to John.

I watched Pop even as I started eating. He had grabbed a bunch of napkins at the condiments table on our way to the booth. He fiddled with them, then arranged his dishes, then—well, I'm not sure what all he did, but it took several minutes before he finally filled his fork with food. He was just about to take his first bite when I announced, "OK, Pop, we're done eating. Let's go!"

He froze, then without raising his head, gave me one of "those" looks. John and I cracked up.

"You can just go on without me," he gruffed, and finished the fork-trip to his mouth. But he really wasn't very hungry—gave me half his salad, saved the cornbread for the birds, left most of his food uneaten, then reached for his pie.

"Uh-uh," I scolded. "You didn't clean your plate, so you can't have dessert." Again, "that" look. He allowed as how he could eat his pie if he wanted to.

Actually, he didn't finish that either. He touched an area above his right ear and said it hurt when he chewed. On the way back to Mayberry, he touched the same area and said it hurt only when he was lying in bed—hurt badly enough that he even asked for an aspirin last night.

Then he mentioned a sore spot where his new dentures were pressing too hard. I'm guessing the pain in his head is associated with the problem inside his mouth. I'll call the dentist tomorrow and get him in for an adjustment.

Poor Pop. It's depressing for him when he can't enjoy his food.

Monday, April 30:

Problems

Kellie called this morning; she suspected the urine around Pop's toilet contained blood. Obviously his aim isn't accurate. (I once asked John how men can miss as big a target as a toilet bowl. He said, "At least I keep it in the bathroom." Thanks, John.)

I went over to check it out. Yep, it looked reddish-orange to me. Called the doc's office and they worked him in. When Dr. Easy-To-Look-At came into the exam room, Pop said, "Oh, I couldn't remember which doctor you were."

I turned to him and said, "He's the cute one!" We both smiled at Dr. A, who kept his eyes on the monitor screen while he recorded Pop's symptoms. He didn't respond except to grin and turn red.

Anyway, it's a bladder infection. Dr. A gave him enough antibiotic samples to knock it out.

I told him about the pain along the right side of Pop's head when he ate or lay down. Dr. A said if the dentist didn't think the new dentures were the problem, then we were to get back to him immediately. It could possibly be temporal arteritis (not arthritis)—an inflammation of a cranial artery, which could be serious.

Aside from all this, I've been battling Medicare for nine months and don't even have a baby to show for it—just a pain in my....

I've been trying to get them to send a No Pay Summary Notice that I can file with Pop's supplemental insurance. We know Medicare won't pay any part of the Mayberry bills, but someone at his secondary insurance said they might cover part of them because he's there as a result of his car wreck—but they'll process a claim only after they receive a refusal from Medicare, which is what I've been trying to get. I've done everything Medicare told me to do. The stack of paperwork is four inches high—literally—and now they say I need to file a UB-92 form which was NEVER mentioned before, which Medicare says it doesn't have, Mayberry doesn't have, the AMA has but sells only in packages of a thousand, and the woman at the local hospital said she can't give me one, which made me start to cry out of complete frustration, which made her transfer me to her supervisor who wasn't there, so I left a voice mail and started crying again, and it's no small wonder she hasn't called me back.

I've been feeling overwhelmed recently, and now I'm worried about Pop. It's like I'm being sucked down into a whirlpool. Or maybe it's just the toilet flushing.

Friday, May 4:

One year ago today

Can you believe it's been a whole year since Pop wrecked his car? Where *has* the time gone?

So what's it been like this last year?

Well, for Pop I'm pretty sure it's been painful—physically and emotionally—in addition to being frightening, depressing, nostalgic, relaxing, comforting, and a vast relief being able to hand over responsibilities that were becoming too much for him. Mostly I think he's content.

You may have noticed I seldom refer to John, his feelings about his dad, or how his dad's dependency affects him. That's because mostly I tell stories about when just Pop and I are together. But John tells me that sometimes he feels good about a visit with his dad; other times he feels frustrated and angry. He's also been recognizing how much like his dad he is. He's proud of the good similarities—hard-working and faithful, to mention two. And he's working to change the tendencies he doesn't like—indecisiveness and procrastination to mention two of those. I'm not real crazy about those tendencies either.

So what's this past year been like for me? Nothing like I expected—or feared. I've been busy and challenged by the handling of two households. I'm frequently exhausted. I get angry when it seems like I'm not getting any cooperation or support from either man. I feel neglected when John spends too much time with his dad—which is kind of funny because I spend more time with Pop than he does, but it's most often when John is at work anyway.

And even though that all sounds negative, I have mostly enjoyed being with Pop. He can be charming, funny, appreciative and quite philosophical at times. Nothing much seems to faze him. I'm usually going at a frantic, full-speed-ahead pace, so when I'm with him and have to slow down, I often find it restful—although admittedly it can also be frustrating and aggravating. Still, he has a gentleness that makes him a pleasure to be with.

This past year hasn't been all peachy keen and bowls of cherries and chestnuts roasting. Sometimes it's been the pits, the bowl has shattered, and the nuts have burned. If Pop were actually living in our tiny house with us, I might have wrapped his walker around his neck by now—or he around mine! But he's not. He's just a mile up the road.

I sometimes think of Mayberry Homes as a miracle place. By having him close, yet not in my hip pocket, I've truly been able to enjoy Pop. I do love that man. I'm glad he's here.

Monday, May 7:
Good news, bad news—and worse news

When Dr. B checked Pop's dentures last week, he said they didn't need adjusting, and that the pain was too high up the side of his head to have anything to do with them anyway. I called Dr. A's and arranged for Pop to go in for a blood test that wouldn't positively diagnose *for* temporal arteritis, but it would at least tell us if he didn't have it.

The good news is he does not have it. The blood test is negative. So what's causing his pain?

I don't know, but the bad news is he might have hepatitis.

Cortney called us Saturday to report Pop's face had a yellow tinge to it. John noticed it when they drove around town on Sunday. Then Kellie called early this morning to say his urine was orange-y red again, plus his whole body was yellow.

As soon as Dr. A's office opened, I left a message asking what to do, gave them my home and cell phone numbers, ran some errands, then stopped in to see Pop for myself. He was definitely jaundiced.

"Hey, Pop, can you sing for me?"

"What?" he said, confused.

"You're as yellow as a canary. Can you sing like one, too?" He grunted a half-laugh.

He said he felt OK, but was tired since he hadn't slept well. "My right arm itched so bad it kept me awake." He pulled back his sleeve to show me—he'd scratched it raw.

I went home and called Dr. A's again. Managed to talk with his nurse, who spoke with the doc, who said to bring Pop in right then for more blood work, and he would come out to the waiting room to take a look at him in-between patients.

After the lab took blood and urine samples, I went in search of the nurse to let her know we were there. I almost bumped bodies with the doc himself as he came out of an exam room. He grinned at me and asked if Pop glowed in the dark.

"No, but he looks like a canary," I chirped. (Yeah, I know— too cute.)

He came out to the waiting room a couple of minutes later and squatted down next to Pop. "Yep, he's definitely yellow." A tech handed doc the test results. He made a sound that didn't mean good news. Not only did Pop still have a bladder infection, but there was bilirubin—which has something to do with the liver—in his urine, which is why Dr. A thinks it's probably hepatitis.

He ordered another lab test to check specifically for it. Meanwhile, Dr. A suggested an over-the-counter antihistamine for the itching. He also suggested isolating Pop as much as possible in case he's contagious. Oh dear.

Wednesday, May 9:

Quarantined

Pop's been quarantined for three days now, and he looks like he's shrinking into himself. He's feeling blue and misses socializing with the ladies. Miss Bess has been flinging his birdseed since he's not even allowed on the porch. He also couldn't take his bath today.

"A-ha! The truth is out now," I teased. "You're doing this just to get out of taking a bath, aren't you." He chuckled half-heartedly.

"I'd be willing to take one when I feel better." Man, he must be feeling puny because that doesn't sound like him at all. I've explained that he might have hepatitis and what it is, but all he wants to know is can they give him some medicine to make him well.

The hepatitis test results aren't in yet, but Dr. A wanted Pop back at the lab this morning to have blood drawn for a hepatic function panel—he wants to see what's going on with the liver.

Mona had already asked me to work today, so I called to let her know I'd be late but would be there ASAP—and wouldn't you know: any time you're in a hurry, that's when you're delayed. Even though I'd called him, Pop wasn't completely dressed when I got to

Mayberry. When he was finally ready, it was a slow journey down the sidewalk to get to my car.

At the doc's office, the only handicapped parking space available was the furthest spot from the front door, plus it forced Pop to step up a curb and practically into some bushes in order to get to the sidewalk—not real convenient for the handicapped if you ask me—but no one did.

When we finally made it inside, only one person was processing people—and we were third in line. We got the OK to go back to the lab waiting room—and four people were ahead of us there. Of course, once they got him in the lab chair, it didn't take long to draw the blood.

Dr. A wasn't in today, but I asked the desk clerk to have one of the other doctors call me at work with the results. A lot of people were being affected by Pop's illness, and we needed to know something as quickly as possible.

Well, a doctor did call, but she didn't know exactly what it was I wanted. Uh-h—lab test results. She didn't have them; she'd call me back. She didn't.

I called again when I got home and was finally put through to a nurse. All she could tell me was hepatitis was contagious during the first two to three weeks after it's contracted—before any symptoms appear. Supposedly, now that Pop's jaundiced, he's not contagious.

"Just how contagious is it though?" I asked the nurse. "Could any of the ladies have been infected by picking up a tissue or napkin he had used?" Possible, but unlikely.

She said hepatitis is a fecal-oral virus, meaning it's contracted when something contaminated with virus-containing fecal matter touches the mouth. Ick. She also said hepatitis is not uncommon in "institutional" settings. Mayberry is so squeaky clean I can't believe he could have contracted it there.

Three weeks ago Pop used a public restroom and could have picked up the virus from touching sink faucets or the door handle. A month ago he was in Tyler with John. He could have picked it up at a rest area or any other place there.

It's disgusting how often people don't wash their hands after using the toilet or after changing a baby, spreading—crap—everywhere. I also think it's gross when people lick their fingers before counting out bills, and it totally gags me when a cashier licks her fingers then opens up a plastic bag—which she then tries to hand to me with her spit all over it. Major Yuck!

However, I am perfectly willing to let Charlie share an ice cream cone with me. Nothing gross about that at all!

Thursday, May 10:

Grrrrr!

OK, the latest news is Pop doesn't have any type of hepatitis. One of Dr. A's nurses called me at work this afternoon. I asked her three times to repeat the information, and three times I asked her, "Are you *sure*?" She confirmed each time that the test showed he doesn't have Type A, B or C hepatitis.

John and I are both relieved that he doesn't, and angry that he had to have all those blood tests because we were told he did—but now Dr. A thinks it may be the Epstein Barr syndrome, which is similar to mononucleosis, the "kissing disease." He doesn't really know. Talk about not getting a definitive answer!

The nurse also said Pop should stop taking the antibiotic for his bladder infection in case the test readings were being affected by it. I objected because you aren't supposed to stop antibiotic treatment midstream. She insisted that's what Dr. A wanted.

Then she asked if I wanted to bring Pop in on Monday. I explained that we'd better have an appointment sooner than that because I wanted some answers *now*. He had already been in quarantine for too long, and I was damned if he was going to be confined over the weekend without good reason. Suddenly there was a 10 a.m. available tomorrow.

I hung up, then called Dianne at Mayberry to let her know Pop didn't have hepatitis, although we still didn't know what he *did* have. By the way, the ladies know he doesn't feel well, of course, but not what's wrong. Actually we don't know either.

He was unshaved and still in his robe when I got there late this afternoon to take the antibiotics out of his meds box—the staff isn't allowed to do it. He's obviously depressed, his voice sounds shaky, his appetite is off, and he looks frail. His confinement is really getting to him.

It's getting to me, too. Between the stress of Pop's illness, not sleeping well, working a lot recently which means the house is a big mess and paperwork is piling up—well, there are just too many demands on my time. Anybody got a few extra hours a day they can give me?

Anyway, I'm sorry I took up the "Wolf!" cry, but my cute Dr. A led me astray. Baa-a-a!

Friday, May 11:

A failure to communicate

Any inflammation of the liver falls under the general category of Hepatitis. Pop's liver is inflamed; therefore he has hepatitis.

When I told Dr. A how upset we were about this hepatitis/not-hepatitis business, he asked if his nurse hadn't read to me what he'd written about the situation—then promptly went to his computer screen and read it again. His rendition cleared up the confusion.

His nurse said Pop didn't have types A, B or C, but she didn't say Epstein Barr was a form of hepatitis, so I thought he didn't have it at all after we'd been told he did. Clear?

It's uncertain at this point exactly what other type of hepatitis he has because those lab tests take longer, and the results aren't in yet.

If he has Epstein Barr, that encompasses several different respiratory-type viruses, including mononucleosis. It takes "intimate" contact to transmit, usually/often through saliva. It can be transmitted by kissing, by touching someone's used Kleenex then not washing the hands before touching the mouth, and even via someone's cold—which totally surprised me, but somehow made sense.

The symptoms for all the different types of hepatitis are the same—fever, jaundice, headache, tiredness, loss of appetite, and itching. Not everyone has all the symptoms. Some people don't display any symptoms, but are carriers.

Pop, by the way, has lost twelve pounds since this started, so he definitely has the loss of appetite symptom. I guess this also explains his headaches, itching and tiredness, not to mention the jaundice.

Dr. A said the hepatic function numbers are coming down, which is a good sign. He'll test them again next week.

In the meantime, he recommended that Pop stay confined to his room. Damn.

Tuesday, May 15:

Pop is in the hospital—

And Dr. A is in DEEP SH*T.

It's 4 a.m. right now. We've been in the Emergency Room for the last ten hours.

The first thing both the ER nurse and doctor asked was: "Has he had an ultrasound?"

"No." They did an ultrasound.

Pop has gallstones and "sludge."

He's never had hepatitis. He's never been contagious.

He spent the last nine days in isolation for nothing.

When I talked to Dr. A's nurse earlier today—I mean yesterday, I guess—and was told Pop's tests were negative for all four Epstein Barr viruses, I asked what other tests could be run because we had to have some answers. She asked Dr. A, who said, "No other tests at this time, but keep him quarantined." For the rest of his life? Come on.

Then late this—I mean—yesterday afternoon Dianne called and said she had talked with the owner of Mayberry, and while they had tried to work with us, they were violating their license by continuing to keep Pop there without knowing if he was contagious or not. They're not set up to handle a continuing quarantine situation. She was sorry, but he had to leave immediately. She suggested we take him to the emergency room.

We didn't know what else to do, so that's what we did.

Was there any excuse for Dr. A overlooking something that now seems obvious? Gallstones blocking a bile duct.

Pop's been through all this for nothing. Mayberry's been through all this for nothing. John and I have been through all this for nothing.

I know I've kidded around about how cute the doc is, but I wouldn't have continued taking Pop to him if I hadn't thought he was good. I am so angry and disappointed that he made such a stupid mistake. *How* could he have missed this?

later Tuesday, May 15:

Just quickly for now—

because I need to go lie down for awhile before John and I go back to the hospital. One-and-a-half hours of sleep just doesn't cut it.

Pop is having an endoscopic procedure around 5 p.m. They want to remove some stones from his bile duct before they remove his gall bladder tomorrow.

Your concerned e-mails are very much appreciated. I'll respond when I can. Life has turned upside down these last couple of days.

Endoscopy, by the way, is when they put a camera down your throat so they can look at your insides from the inside.

More later ...

Tuesday evening, May 15:

Crap—

Pop may have pancreatic cancer.

They're going to do a CT-scan-directed biopsy tomorrow.

The surgeon who did the endoscopy said the pancreatic duct was involved somehow—and based on his experience, that is almost always indicative of cancer.

Wednesday, May 16:

What's going on with Pop

Late last night Dr. Z cheerfully (it seemed) told John and me that when a pancreatic duct looked the way Pop's did, it almost always indicated pancreatic cancer.

Pop was moved out of ER and into a room. We went in to say "good night" to him, trying not to look as stricken as we felt, because we decided to wait until we had all gotten a couple hours sleep before we told him. No point in making the bleary-eyed, will-it-ever-be-over ER ordeal even worse than it already was.

Because they had him scheduled for the CT scan with endoscopic needle-biopsy at nine this morning, John made sure he got to the hospital to talk with his dad about Dr. Z's report before they took him down.

I walked Charlie first, then dreading it, went to the hospital. As soon as I walked into his room, Pop told me, "Barbara, you know I have cancer."

"Pop, we don't know that for sure."

A little later he said, "I don't have cancer, do I?" We reminded him that we didn't know yet.

The aides came in and rolled him away. While it's not one hundred percent accurate, the report from yesterday's scan said there was "no visible mass" on the pancreas, which could be good news. The doctor told us folds in the pancreatic duct sometime give the illusion of a mass pushing against it.

In today's procedure, as best I understood it, the hollow endoscopic needle poked a hole through the duct (which is extraordinarily tiny anyway), hit a minute area of pancreas, then sucked in tissue cells through the needle. They also put in a plastic stent to open the duct so the bile can flow again, which will clear up the jaundice.

If the biopsy comes back negative, that's good news, of course, but tempered with the fact that they could have taken "clean" cells and missed cancerous cells right next to them—meaning we still wouldn't know for sure.

If it's negative, they'll go ahead with the gall bladder surgery. If it's positive, well ... we just go from there.

As awful as it was having him thrown out of Mayberry, at least we're close to getting some answers now, even if they might not be answers we want.

The other news is Mayberry is ready for Pop to come "home," cancer or no cancer. They've thoroughly cleaned his room and opened the window to air it out. Plus Gabriella's been using a fabric cleaner on his recliner—she scrubs on it every chance she gets.

After the procedure, when Pop was back in his bed, he started talking to John and me, rambling along, I think, as a way of processing and dealing with this newest "car wreck." Actually, he's handling it better than we are.

Pop's a Christian. He said he knows he'll get to see his wife and his parents again, and he'd be happy about that. "I've had a good life. If it's my time to die, I'm at peace with it, and I'm willing to go.

However," he emphasized with a smile, "if it's *not* my time, I'm quite willing to stick around for awhile."

By the way, I called Dr. A's office yesterday. The receptionist could tell I was upset, which is an understatement if I ever wrote one. Dr. A called me back almost immediately.

I was too tired to be careful about what I said, and I barely took a breath when I told him we'd just spent ten hours in the ER because Mayberry had kicked out Pop, that we'd been asked immediately if he'd had an ultrasound, and we had to say, "No, Dr. A never ordered one," that we were angry because Pop had spent nine days in isolation for no reason, that we thought he was a good doctor—but *how* could he have missed gallstones? Why hadn't he ordered an ultrasound? I was only half-kidding when I wailed, "I thought you were perfect! I had you on a pedestal!"

To his credit, he didn't get defensive. He apologized, then explained that Pop didn't have any pain or tenderness in that area. (My Mom had a lot of pain when she had gallstones.) The liver function numbers had been high and were coming down, which was very typical of a viral infection. He said that sometimes older people don't exhibit the same symptoms as younger people, and he would remember that from now on.

Well, even though I had to "confront" him, the hospital Admitting Doctor had already saved his bacon. She'd spoken with us the night/morning she admitted Pop, wanting to know if he had any special problems before he underwent gall bladder surgery. When I told her about the hepatitis fiasco, she said Dr. A was a good doctor; yes, he probably should have ordered an ultrasound, but since Pop didn't have any symptoms except jaundice, it's not surprising that he didn't suspect gallstones immediately.

I expected John would want to "fire" the doc, but his response was, "If God can give someone a second chance, I guess I can, too." Pop likes Dr. A. Maybe I'm a fool, but I still think he's a good doctor—and it has nothing to do with his being cute. I'm disillusioned because he isn't perfect, but then I'm not either. (I am, however, Saint Flossie!)

Listen, I gotta tell you: Monday afternoon before we took Pop to the ER, I had to take Charlie to the vet for a problem that may have been triggered by the stress of these last three days. He's a mama's dog, and I haven't been able to pay much attention to him, plus I'm sure he's been sensitive to John's and my emotional upheaval.

The vet had to stick a long probe up Charlie's hiney to get a sample. Sometime during the wee small hours in the ER, an aide came into the exam room and stuck a probe up Pop's fanny to get a sample.

I went back in after she left and told him, "If it makes you feel any better, I took Charlie to the vet this afternoon, and he had a probe stuck up his butt like you did just now—" and spreading my hands apart to illustrate the length, added, "only Charlie's probe was a *whole* lot longer than yours." Pop guffawed. Yes—guffawed.

One more thing: We've kept Mark updated since this situation started. Mark and Pop look a lot alike, and both love playing practical jokes, but otherwise their personalities are polar opposites.

Pop was the serious-minded, dutiful child who learned about hard work at a very early age, who was discharged from the Army Air Corps because, during WWII, two sons of a widowed mother couldn't be in service at the same time. The farthest he ever got from home was when he and Mother Pat went to Alaska to see John after he joined the Air Force and was stationed in Anchorage.

Mark, three years younger, was the wild child, the cut-up, the one with no responsibilities at home, the one who traveled all over the world when he was in the service. He's had stomach and prostate cancers, and he's still around. Point being: The Blanks Boys are tough old coots. But Mark is still scared for his brother.

Thursday, May 17:
'round and 'round we go...

Dr. Z, the one who first suspected cancer, was supposed to be making his hospital rounds, but he must have been 'round about somewhere else, because he wasn't around Pop at all today. More on that later.

First, because hospitals love shuffling people, they moved Pop to a room right across from the nurse's station. The orange dot on the name tag outside his new room means he's considered a "falling risk."

Second, the Care Group at John's church sent him a vase of assorted flowers and festive balloons. Pastor Keith and Assistant Pastor Susan came to see him yesterday, too.

Third, the hospital has kept Pop in bed for four days, and after what now totals thirteen days of inactivity, he's gotten weak and really is a falling risk. They won't let John or me walk him, so yesterday I asked about exercise for him—without results. Today I got pushy about it. They found a doctor to prescribe physical therapy, which means Pop will walk the hall with a therapist once a day. That's all insurance will allow, but it's better than nothing.

Fourth, I called Dr. A's office this morning and left a message— partly to say we were OK with him continuing as Pop's primary physician, partly to ask about the second lab report concerning liver function tests. Since I was about to leave for the hospital, I gave them my cell phone number, forgetting John had taken it with him.

So when John answered, Dr. A probably thought, "Oh great, now *he's* going to yell at me!" He told John that he'd lost sleep over Pop's misdiagnosis, and that he'd been praying about it. He said he learned something, and he'd be a better doctor because of it. John believed him. I do, too.

Fifth, John called me early this evening to say they'd taken Pop off the I.V. antibiotic for his bladder infection, per Dr. D, who is going to do the gall bladder surgery. (He's the one who did his hernia surgery last August.) John also said Dr. Z still hadn't shown up.

Sixth, we spent most of today (taking turns) waiting to hear about the biopsy results from yesterday's procedure. The Admitting Doctor finally came to the room around 3 p.m. She said she had just talked with the lab. There weren't any results. They hadn't taken any tissue for biopsy. Apparently Dr. Z's order had been to focus the CT scan on the pancreas and take tissue from the "mass." When they didn't see one, they didn't take tissue. Even so, stricture of this duct is almost always caused by a mass pressing against it. Just because the scan didn't see it doesn't mean it's not there.

She didn't know what Dr. Z planned to do. He might take tissue from the "strictured" (like a straw squeezed closed) pancreatic duct, but it is almost certain—get this—it is almost certain they will *not* remove Pop's gall bladder after all. The bile duct isn't blocked, so it didn't cause the jaundice. He's not in pain; there's no infection. They'll probably leave it alone. (By the way, the "sludge" I mentioned before is their word for thick gunk (bile?) that accumulates in the gall bladder and can eventually become stones.)

So, essentially we've lost another week and all we know for sure is Pop has gallstones. Limbo sucks.

Still, he feels pretty good. He ate most of his breakfast, but less than half his lunch. He stuck his fork in the fried chicken and asked me, "Is this the tail of a chicken?" He paused, giving me a sideways grin. "At least I think that's what it's called."

"Pop, do you mean you're eating a chicken's butt?"

He laughed out loud. "Guess so."

After he'd taken a few bites he said, "I can't eat all of this. Do you think Charlie would care what part of the chicken he's eating?"

"Not in the least."

It's after eight now, and John just got home. Dr. Z didn't show up again, and John is furious. He left a message at the nurse's station saying Dr. Z had better talk to us tomorrow morning. We're fed up with him and his insensitivity.

Friday, May 18:

Pop is back at Mayberry!

We never did see Dr. Z—the jerk—but Dr. D came in this morning and started doctor-talking to us. I interrupted him, saying, "Draw us a picture, please." While he sketched organs, he reverted to normal-person speech. Here's what I understood:

There's a duct that comes from the gall bladder, and another one that comes from the pancreas. They join together as they enter the duodenum (upper part of the small intestine.) That juncture is compressed, which was why the bile acids got stuck and backed up, which was why Pop got jaundiced. (His color is almost normal now, thanks to that plastic stent.)

The bad news is the ducts are strictured, which indicates cancer. There's a lesion on one of those ducts, which indicates cancer. Jaundice without pain is a pretty positive indicator of cancer.

If it's cancer, it's most likely a type that grows really fast. There is also a "spot" on Pop's liver, which could mean the cancer has already metastasized (spread). There's a very small possibility the ducts are strictured due to inflammation caused by irritation from gallstone particles, which could cause pancreatitis, which isn't good, but it's better than cancer.

Dr. D thinks Pop should go to a specialist who would evaluate the CT and ultrasound films. Pop insisted that whatever John and I decided was all right with him. It's nice that he has that much confidence in us, but we don't want that kind of responsibility. It's *his* life. But with his approval, we opted for the specialist.

133

I told Dr. D that I wanted hard copies of all the hospital reports from ER to now. Almost everyone we've dealt with has been great except one—a nurse with a bad attitude who seemed exceedingly unhappy with me. Maybe she didn't like that I'd been pushy about getting exercise for Pop? Maybe making copies was too much extra work for her? Maybe she didn't like me exerting Pop's patient rights?

I don't know. I didn't care. She tried to refuse my request, saying "legally" Dr. D had to OK us getting copies.

"He already has," I told her, "and *legally* we are entitled to all these medical records." The point here is: ALWAYS ask for copies of your lab work and written diagnoses. I just quickly went through the paperwork a few minutes ago, and have already seen—if not outright mistakes—then inaccuracies. The Admitting Doctor recorded Pop had *not* lost weight and still had an appetite—after I clearly told her early Tuesday a.m. that Pop had lost over 12 lbs and had *no* appetite. Seems minor maybe, but maybe not.

Anyway, before I got there today, Pop had an actual shower instead of a bed-bath. The aide slapped baby powder all over him, put him in a clean gown, and sat him down in a vinyl chair until the bed linens were changed.

He and John were watching TV when I arrived. I used wet paper towels to wipe off the visible powder on the chair seat before sitting down, not realizing more was hiding in the cushion crevices. When I stood up—I wanted coffee—the seat of my pants was covered with powder; John saw it as I passed in front of him. He stopped me, and started brushing the powder off with his hand.

Pop watched a minute then asked, "What is John doing to you?"

"He's playing with my butt, Pop." He began chuckling. "Want me to bend over and tell him to kiss it?"

Pop threw back his head and roared. Oh, it was good hearing him laugh!

So, he was discharged this afternoon. Flowers and "Welcome Back" balloons were in his room at Mayberry. His recliner was so clean it looked practically new.

Several of the ladies had been watching for him—they opened the front door as he was getting out of the car.

You think that man won't be purely spoiled?

Wednesday, May 23:
Pop's appetite and appointment

He called on Sunday, his voice a little shaky. He said he hadn't eaten anything all day, but now a Whataburger sounded good. He hated to bother us, but if John was coming over later, could he bring him one, if it wasn't too much trouble?

"How about if you go to the burger rather than the burger come to you?" John asked. Pop must have liked the idea, because he was waiting on the porch when John drove up.

Today I called the cancer specialist. The appointment is next Tuesday afternoon. I'll pick up the ultrasound and CT scan films from the Garland hospital so we can take them with us.

Ya know, a year ago I never would have thought a car wreck could be a blessing—especially since I don't generally even use that word—but that's what it took to move Pop up here.

Out of the wreckage a relationship has developed that Pop and I wouldn't have had otherwise, and that is definitely a blessing. I can't begin to tell you how grateful I am for that. John and Pop have grown closer, too, and that's good.

Poor John. He had signed up to take four days off last week—fortuitously as it turned out—but he sure hadn't planned to spend his entire vacation at the hospital. Nothing I wanted to do around here got done either, and I don't even get the fun of bellyaching about it.

Wednesday, May 30:
Meeting with the cancer specialist

We met with Dr. S yesterday afternoon. He said it's almost one-hundred-percent certain it's pancreatic cancer. They look for six signs. Pop has all six: painless jaundice, bouts of diarrhea, loss of appetite, weight loss, intense itching—and something else I can't think of right now.

CT scans generally show pancreatic tumors only after they've grown fairly large. That means Pop's tumor is probably no bigger than a thumb nail, but removing it would still require extensive surgery because portions of several major organs would have to be removed, too.

Problems with resectioning (reconnecting) those organs often occur afterward. Pop might not make it through post-op or the recovery period. If he survived, he'd be diabetic, and his quality of life wouldn't ever return to its current level.

Not only would he have to pass the pre-op physical, but that spot on his liver would have to be biopsied, because if the cancer has spread, all bets are off.

Pop says he doesn't want surgery.

Focalized radiation would be the other option, but it would only slow down the cancer, not eradicate it. When Dr. S told us about all the side effects, Pop joked that at least wouldn't have to worry about hair loss. This option is on hold, because a lot will depend on what they see on Friday.

Dr. S wants a Dr. N to do an endoscopic-guided ultrasound to try to locate the exact position of the tumor and take tissue for biopsy. Either it will be malignant...or not. Dr. N would also replace the fragile plastic stent with a metal one to prevent a reoccurrence of the jaundice.

Before we left the exam room Dr. S prescribed digestive enzymes for Pop to take with each meal. Because his pancreas isn't functioning properly, his body isn't absorbing nutrients, which is why he's losing weight.

Pop and John went back to the waiting room—actually they exited to the restroom—while I stayed behind to get instructions from the nurse. Since Dr. S was standing right next to me, I choked out the question none of us had asked earlier.

He confirmed what Dr. D told us: Pop's looking at months, not years.

It was a quiet ride back to Mayberry. Pop didn't want to go to a cafeteria with us for supper, but said, "I wouldn't mind if you brought me some more Pringles." Later that night Nancy Lee called us to say Pop had called her, cried and almost hung up on her, then cried some more. I guess his diagnosis was sinking in.

This morning I took him to the optician to have his glasses adjusted. On the way inside, he had to hitch up his jeans—they're so loose his belt is cinched up as far as it can go.

"I think you should change your name to Droopy Drawers, Pop," I said.

He gave it some thought.

"Would folks call me D.D. instead of J.D.?"

Pop needed to lose weight, but not like this. Jeez.

Friday, June 1:

Pop's biopsy

Even though his biopsy wasn't scheduled until 11 a.m., we picked up Pop about ten, his stomach rumbling from lack of breakfast. We wanted to allow plenty of time since we didn't know where we were going—well, we knew which hospital but not how long it would take to get there. Didn't want them to start without Pop after all.

John let us out at the entrance, then went to park. Pop and I walked right to the In-Patient Admissions Office, finding it exactly where I was told it would be. Normally this endoscopic procedure is considered day surgery, but they wanted him processed as an in-patient in case there were complications, and he had to stay overnight.

I signed him in. We sat in Presbyterian's tiny waiting room for less than ten minutes before we were called into a cubicle to start the Paperwork Polka. We were almost done when John showed up. In spite of my directions—or maybe because of them—he had taken the elevator to the Out-Patient Admissions Office downstairs. Eventually he had to admit to someone that he'd lost his father and his wife, and was redirected upstairs. Don't think I won't rub that in!

Anyway, the paperwork man led us to the third floor and left us in a "prep" room. A nurse gave Pop a gown and told him to strip down to his skivvies.

After the aide rolled him away, John and I were shown to a small, private GI (Gastrointestinal) Waiting Room, which we appreciated because the big Out-patient Waiting/Registration Room down the hall was noisy and packed with people. Still, I walked to it three times because that's where the coffee was, and just past *it* were the restrooms. Made it convenient to empty and fill up on the same trip.

Waiting rooms are hard places to be in…because you have to wait. One man was waiting to find out why his mother was having trouble swallowing. He got a report and left. A woman came in and briefly spoke with someone on her cell phone, saying her dad was being worked on. When I glanced at her, I could see she was trying not to cry. On impulse I went over and hugged her. She said her dad had rectal bleeding, and she was scared. She talked to me until her doctor came in. I moved away to sit with John again, but blatantly eaves-dropped until hearing her dad didn't have cancer but something else that was treatable. I smiled and gave her a thumbs-up.

Not long after she left, Dr. N came in. He, like Dr. S, talked to us openly and directly, just as we'd requested.

First he said he'd taken four tissue samples, which caused some bleeding that obscured the site, so he hadn't put in the metal stent after all. Then he told us, "The ultrasound very clearly shows a tumor one inch long and just under a half-inch wide." It was positioned at the juncture of the pancreatic and bile ducts.

Dr. N explained that there are different kinds of pancreatic cancers. A tumor inside the duct usually grows slowly. Tumors in or on the pancreas itself grow at different rates for different people. Tumors that grow where Pop's is located are the most aggressive. Those cancers can grow to golf-ball size in one month and to tennis-ball size in two. That's starting from thumb-nail size.

He didn't completely rule out a benign tumor, but his experience has been that tumors in that position in someone Pop's age are usually malignant. They take tissue for biopsy just to remove any lingering doubt. Results should be back by Tuesday or Wednesday.

Whether he chooses radiation or not, Dr. N suggested we "retain" an oncologist since they are quite adept at managing pain. (Pop watched his mother die an agonizing death from ovarian cancer. Pain is the only thing he fears.)

After Dr. N left, I put my needlepoint back in my totebag, not looking at John because I was desperately trying not to cry. That lasted about ten seconds before I started sobbing, which broke John's restraint. Thank goodness the room was empty except for us because we sat there hugging each other and blubbering.

We finally pulled ourselves together. "Showtime," I said, and grimaced. Dr. N had directed us to a different waiting area, where we waited for Pop to be moved out of Recovery—and into a different room, of course.

He was alert when they brought him in. Both Dr. N and the nurse anesthesiologist came to check on him. He listened patiently to the news that he had a tumor, that it was probably malignant, that he probably had less than a year, and then he asked, "When can I get something to eat? I'm *hungry*!" Made all of us laugh. Trust Pop to put important things first.

By then it was about 4 p.m. John went home to let out Charlie before he exploded. Someone brought Pop a bowl of chicken noodle soup, crackers, and apple juice. He couldn't get it down fast enough. After he ate, I sat on the edge of the bed and encouraged him to talk.

"What was John like as a baby?"

"He was a good boy. His mother worshipped him." He got teary-eyed.

"Did you ever change his diapers?"

Pop laughed. "No, I don't believe I did."

He expressed concern about John's job—he wasn't in trouble for taking off so much time, was he?

"No, he's taking vacation time—he has plenty of it."

Then he thought maybe after he died John could retire on what he would inherit. Not even close, but I didn't say that.

I shook my head. "Do you remember after you first retired how Mother wanted to kill you?"

His whole face cracked into a smile. He ducked his head and laughed, then admitted, "Yes, I remember."

"Well, Pop, that's what I'd have to do if John retired now—kill him."

He wanted to know what he weighed. 179.2 pounds. He grinned, and allowed as how he probably didn't have to be careful about how many snacks he ate any more.

"Your belt is cinched up to where it can't be cinched any tighter. You can have all the Little Debbie's, Pringles and ice cream you want until you get to the other end of your belt again."

I was pretty sure he knew nothing about anatomy—except the "important" stuff—so I asked if he had understood all the talk about pancreatic ducts and gall bladders.

"Well, sure," he started to say, then changed it to, "No, not really."

So, like Dr. D had done, I drew a very simple diagram, tried to explain about the organs involved with simple analogies that he essentially understood, showed him where the tumor was, then went over everything with him a second time to reinforce it since his memory is so bad.

About then an aide came in to help Pop to the bathroom. I asked her if he could have more soup since he was still hungry. In fact, could we possibly have two bowls of soup—one for me, too, because I was starving. "Can I have some extra crackers?" Pop chimed in. Sure could. Yea! We ate our soup, and shared the crackers.

Shortly after John got back to the hospital, Pop was discharged. He had missed supper at Mayberry by that time, but I'd called earlier and asked Yvette, the night shift lady, to save some for him, which she did. Pop finally got his first real meal of the day. He was a happy man.

Saturday, June 2:

Pop and Faucet Man

Some idiot invented the washerless faucet, which means when it starts leaking, you have to replace the whole thing—not just the washers—which means what used to be a simple chore has become a major job.

Today John played plumber, going outside every so often to turn the water Off or On, but mostly clanging around under the kitchen sink. I kept him company, diligently working on some rubberstamped cards in my "office," trying to coincide the after-effects of my coffee drinking with water-On times, pointedly not offering to help (unless asked) because past experience has shown that to be the wiser course.

My office is our small dining area, because years ago I replaced the dining table (which mostly functioned as a desk without drawers anyway) with a real desk and a computer table. John and I don't entertain, although we *are* rather entertaining—kind of like Laurel and Hardy but only because we fall one Stooge short of being The Three, so we don't miss the dining table at all.

John clanged and sweated; I stamped. Then Pop called. Was John coming over after lunch? They had plans to drive around.

"Yes, just as soon as he finishes changing out the faucet."

"Oh. OK."

Ten minutes later he called again, having forgotten he'd already called. I reminded him about the faucet. Fifteen minutes later he called again, wondering if John was done yet.

"No, but he has to go look for a part he thinks he needs, so how about if he brings you over here on his way back?"

"That'd be all right."

I'd seen Pop yesterday and he looked okay, but today his lips looked bruised, and he seemed fragile. He and Charlie sat outside on the patio, watching the birds until Spike, the kitten from next door, delighted him by paying a visit.

Inside, I finished my cards and spread them out over the desk so the ink could dry.

John kept plugging away under the sink, until finally, forgetting he hadn't turned the water to Off again, he unscrewed one of the new faucet handles to check something.

Can you say "water pressure?" The geyser reached my desk and splattered on the ink. Instant watercolor. Thanks, John.

Late this afternoon, he finally decided the faucet we'd bought wasn't going to work with our sink, so he put the old one back on. He and Pop went for their drive.

Before John ever got started this morning, I reminded him what a job it had been the last time he changed a faucet. I *tried* suggesting we call a plumber.

"It'll save you a lot of aggravation," I said.

But No-o-o-o-o! He chose to spend his whole Saturday with the cabinet floor wedged into his back and plumber's putty falling on his face. Men!

The faucet still drips, by the way. And the hot water handle turns backwards.

Sunday, June 3:

Pop right now

Thank you all for your concerned e-mails, but please remember that Pop is still doing OK. We don't know how long the good months will last, but when John took him riding around again this afternoon, they stopped at Whataburger for supper. For now, his appetite is better than it was.

I do know I'm thankful so many of you gave me positive feedback every time I posted stories about Pop, which meant I continued to write them ... which means I'll be able to look back later and remember those little moments that usually slip easily from memory. Too often you only realize in hindsight how special those moments were.

So many of you have "adopted" Pop as your own. He couldn't have a better family.

Tuesday, June 5:

Pop's biopsy report

Dr. N called.
It's malignant.
The most aggressive kind.

Wednesday, June 6:

Pop takes advantage

Pop didn't have a bath on Monday, even though he needed one. He talked himself out of it by telling Margaret, "I have cancer. I don't have to take a bath if I don't want to."

He didn't say it as a sympathy ploy, mind you. He just didn't want a bath and was wielding any excuse he could come up with to get out of it. Margaret let him win that time, but she threatened him with a thorough scrubbing on Wednesday.

I picked up some Fig Newtons while I was out today, then stopped to see him on my way home. Margaret had been as good as her word. Pop pointed to his head and bellyached, "Do you see what that old woman did to me? She scrubbed off half my hair."

Tuesday, June 12:

A tale of three days

John and Pop drove to Longview on Sunday to have lunch with Mark. Pop wouldn't talk to his brother about his cancer. He said Mark wasn't feeling well and didn't want to burden him.

After lunch, John took his dad to Nancy Lee's. He hadn't seen her since before Christmas, although he'd called her regularly.

Yesterday morning we went to the oncologist's office for the first time—a difficult drive to a depressing destination. It wasn't a long drive, but I teased Pop about Nancy Lee, trying to keep things light. He said they sat on her back porch and talked about old times.

"Did you do any smooching?" I asked him.

"Well, sur-r-r-re!" he said, flashing his new teeth in a big grin.

Well, my initial impressions of Dr. O's whole setup were not good.

First, the waiting room was packed. I figured the doctor was overbooked which would mean a long wait, but shortly after I filled out the forms, we were called in. As we passed through the inner door, we encountered a logjam of people. Not only were patients milling around the check-out desk to our left, but Pop was immediately accosted by a crazed woman who wanted to stick a thermometer in his ear. At the same time, another woman tried to rush him onto the weight scale. Pop and his walker don't maneuver easily, and she was trying to shift him faster than he could shift.

Second, after we were shown to an exam room, an insurance woman bustled in. She wanted to be sure his information was correct, then essentially said, "We're going to get paid no matter what happens to you." *That* didn't sit well with me.

Third, a nurse's assistant came in and wanted to know why he was there. (Hello?) She asked the same questions that were on the forms I'd just filled out—and then she filled out a second form with the same answers. She asked about Pop's medications—which I had just listed, so she pulled *that* form out of the folder she had right in front of her and copied it. Jeez Louise!

Fourth, Dr. O came in, but didn't introduce himself. He asked a couple of questions, then sat with his back to us going through the information Dr. N had sent to him. He yawned twice, and rapidly flapped his legs open and closed—like he was dancing the Charleston sitting down.

As I watched him I thought: How could Dr. A recommend this guy? How fast can we get out of here? Man, we need to find another oncologist.

Then Dr. O turned around and focused completely on Pop. He asked questions; he listened to the answers. Even when I had to fill in details, he tended to keep his eyes on Pop. My opinion of him did a one-eighty.

He said he didn't think surgery was an option—either Pop would die on the table or during recovery. Radiation and chemo, either together or separately, were options, but wouldn't prolong his life by very much. He told us about hospice care, about controlling pain, about making Pop as comfortable as possible during the time remaining.

Dr. O said four to six months. He wanted to start hospice immediately. My mind resisted the information, but Pop said, "I'm a

Christian, and I'm at ease knowing I'll be going Home." Doc said he, too, was a Christian. Pop's face lit up.

"Would you pray for me?" he asked. Dr. O assured him he would.

When the doc got up to leave, he leaned over and gave Pop a hug—a real hug. Then he hugged me and kissed me very lightly on the cheek. It was comforting somehow, and I almost lost it then. Give me clinical and practical and I'm strong; give me kindness and gentleness and I crack.

This afternoon we had a get-acquainted, fill-out-the-forms appointment with Lori, a hospice RN, who was cheerful, organized, informative, matter-of-fact and caring. She read all the paperwork out loud and explained it before Pop signed.

It amazed her that he didn't have any pain, not even from his arthritis; she thought the prognosis time-frame must be wrong. I explained what we'd been told about the aggressiveness of this cancer.

Since Pop's blood pressure was normal, and since he was actually a little dehydrated, Lori called Dr. O and got the OK to discontinue his diuretic. Maybe that will help him not have to get up so often at night—that's still his biggest complaint.

Lori will come at least once a week to monitor him. Pop, who had initially been withdrawn and speaking too quietly, was speaking normally and had perked up considerably by the time she was ready to leave. I think he liked her.

Before I left, he told me he was out of Pringles. "You know the kind I like."

John took some to him tonight. Whatever he wants now ...

Saturday, June 16:
Pop has a procedure, then scares us

To prevent the jaundice from reoccurring, Pop was scheduled to have that metal stent "installed" yesterday. No point in both John and me staying at the hospital all day. We decided he would go on to work after dropping off Pop; I'd follow them in my car, and bring him home afterwards.

Good thing for that decision because when John got to Mayberry, Pop was still nekkid. After he got dressed, they got as far

144

as the car before he had to go back in to use the bathroom. No peeing in the bushes to speed things up this time.

Of course I didn't know all that. I kept looking out the window, watching for them, got impatient and went outside to wait in my car. Sat there a couple of minutes, realized I'd forgotten the insurance info, and ran back inside to get it. That's when John called to say they were actually finally heading my way.

Thinking it would save time (like a minute) if they didn't have to drive all the way back to the house, I drove to the end of our block, turned left and parked in the direction we'd be heading, and watched for them in my rearview mirror. John almost turned at our corner anyway before realizing the crazy woman frantically waving her arm out her car window was me.

John dropped off his dad and his walker at the front entrance of the hospital. He waited there until I parked, then Pop and I walked inside to begin our seven-and-a-half hour adventure.

He checked in; someone led us upstairs to his room; an aide told him to get all nekkid again. "Not his underpants," I protested.

"Yes, those, too." As soon as she left I told him to leave them on. The doctor was going down his throat—why should he have to take off his skivvies? He didn't have to the last time. Sure enough, when the real nurse came in, she said leave them on.

After they took him away, another aide led me to the GI waiting room where Dr. N had broken the cancer confirmation to us. I carted the walker, my totebag with magazines and food, purse, and a water-filled tub containing Pop's teeth. Several people were waiting in the room this time, but they gradually left until only one woman and I remained. I asked if she'd like a cup of coffee—I knew where to get some if she'd watch my stuff (except my purse, of course.) Sounded good to her.

Sounded great to me, too—I needed to unload the two cups I'd had since Pop and I first stepped into the Admissions waiting room. Brought back the coffee and settled in to wait. Dr. N eventually called on the room phone. The plastic stent had been successfully replaced with a metal one.

Those CT and ultrasound films from the Garland hospital were in Dr. N's possession. I asked if he was going to return them himself or give them to me so I could—I felt responsible for them since I'd signed them out. Dr. N had them delivered to me in the waiting room.

He called again later and said they'd be wheeling Pop out of recovery in a couple of minutes, and I could meet them at the elevator. I juggled purse, totebag, walker, huge awkward envelope of x-rays, and that small, covered container of teeth that had to be kept upright and level or it would leak, and walked down the hall. If I'd had to chew gum, too, I probably wouldn't have been able to move.

The restroom was right across from the elevator. I decided I'd better stop to unload that third cup of coffee. Set everything down, set myself down, picked myself and everything else back up, re-balanced, and walked over to the elevator. I waited and waited and waited. No sign of Pop. I was about to go upstairs by myself when a man from the GI waiting room approached and said a nurse had been looking for me.

He offered to take me to her and to carry the walker, so I had to re-balance again. We found the nurse, who carried the walker as she led me upstairs. Apparently they wheeled Pop right past me while I was otherwise Occupied. Either that or I went to the wrong elevator, which was entirely possible.

"Hey, Pop! I thought I'd lost you and didn't know *how* I was going to explain that to your son!"

He grinned, awake and alert, but had his eyes on the aide behind me, who'd come in with chicken noodle soup, crackers and apple juice. Last time they did an endoscopy, he wasn't allowed to eat or drink immediately afterwards. I challenged the aide three times; each time she insisted the doctor said it was OK.

Pop chowed down. He no sooner finished than a nurse came in and spotted the empty dishes.

"Oh no! He wasn't supposed to have anything to eat yet!"

I told her what happened. She said she'd have a word with the aide. Lesson: Never believe food delivery persons in a hospital when you're pretty sure you know better than they do. I told the nurse Pop was part goat, so he'd probably be all right.

He kept the food down just fine, of course, but because the doctor pumps air into the stomach to make it easier to see and maneuver the instruments, Pop belched several times, apologizing after each one.

You should know by now that I occasionally use certain words because he doesn't expect to hear them from me, and it takes him by surprise. Also, I was sitting in a chair near the foot of his bed so not only could we see each other, but I could pat his blanket-covered feet once in awhile.

Well, when he started belching, I assured him it didn't bother me.

"But," I added, "if you even *think* about Farting, you tell me. I'm in your direct line of fire, and I want a chance to get out of the way. Don't you *dare* be like your son who will fart in front of a fan that's aimed in my direction. You warn me so I can go to the other side of the room!"

Pop's eyes and smile had gotten real big the first time I said "fart." By the time I finished my dramatic dissertation, he was shaking with laughter. We both dozed a little after that. When we talked later, he asked me if everything was OK with what they had just done. "I don't have cancer or anything like that?"

Truly, I don't think he forgets, but it may be his way of hoping what he remembers is wrong. "You still have cancer, Pop, but you shouldn't have to go through any more procedures like this."

Eventually I went in search of a nurse to find out when he could go home. One came in, checked his vitals, checked with the doctor, told him to put on his clothes, then told me to let her know when I was going for the car so she could put him in a wheelchair and take him downstairs.

"Let's get you dressed, Pop!"

He asked me to pull his jeans on over his feet and part way up his legs to help him get started. After he got hold of the waistband, I sat on the other side of the bed, my back against his, partly to give him privacy, partly to keep him from toppling backwards as he pulled up his britches.

When he finished dressing, I once again balanced purse, totebag, walker, and envelope of films—but no teeth since they were back in Pop's mouth—which meant I had a finger free to push the elevator button. Got the car, got Pop, got on our way.

"I saw a Braum's when we drove by this morning. Want some ice cream?"

"No, I don't think so," he said. However, when we got close to it, I asked again, and that time he thought a cup of vanilla sounded good. We pulled into the drive-through, ordered, picked up, and I actually turned in the right direction when we left the parking lot and got back on the road.

Unfortunately I also ran a red light two blocks later. I saw it turn red, but it didn't register in my brain or with my foot—that tells you how tired I was. I'm just grateful cross-traffic hadn't started moving yet—and that I didn't get a ticket. We made it back to Mayberry in time for Pop to take a nap before supper.

Well, early this afternoon Cortney called to say he felt hot, couldn't get up by himself, and was so shaky and dizzy he could barely walk.

Oh great. John was helping move cabinets into his church's new building and hadn't taken *his* newly acquired cell phone, which made it totally useless for just this kind of emergency. The air-conditioning repair man had called to say he was on his way to our house. I could have left a note on the door and gone anyway, but instead, I asked Greg-next-door if he'd go find John and tell him he needed to go to his dad.

John called from Mayberry a little later. He'd gotten Pop to lie down, then offered him a glass of Coke, not expecting he'd drink it, but he sucked it down fast. He was incredibly thirsty. John poured some water down him. Pop started feeling better.

Duh! He was dehydrated. He didn't have many fluids yesterday. I asked Cortney to have him drink something whenever she checked on him. He'll do it for her.

June 17: Father's Day

Pop misunderstands

John drove his dad around for a couple of hours this afternoon before they came by the house to pick me up. Pop had the choice of supper at a restaurant or ice cream at Braum's. He said he wasn't very hungry and chose Braum's. He ordered a chocolate milkshake.

John went to get a cup of water, and that's when I thought to tell Pop that a social worker from hospice was coming to see him tomorrow morning.

"There's plenty of time for you to have your bath first," I added, "so don't try to weasel out of it." He smiled, then his face puzzled-up.

"Barbara, isn't hospice for people that don't get well?"

"Yes, Pop," I said, reluctantly. He touched his hand to his chest, where he thinks that metal stent is.

"I thought that 'thing' fixed my problem," he said.

My heart sank into my stomach and my stomach sank to my knees. He had again gotten it into his head that his cancer had been cured.

"No, the stent is just supposed to keep you from becoming jaundiced again."

He sat there, staring at the table, working his mouth a little, processing the information. Oh man, *another* car wreck. The look on his face made me feel lower than scum—reminding him on Father's Day that he has cancer when he thought he was cured.

Then Pop, who often deals with his feelings by submerging them, was OK again. He went back to drinking his milkshake. He didn't say anything to John. (I told him later.)

Pop needed to use the restroom before we left. They walked down the hall, and John pushed open the door. Did the sign say Women? Door closed. Yep: Women. Hmm-m-m...I expected the door to open again immediately, but it didn't. No ladies walked toward the restroom, so I stayed seated.

When they came out, I jabbed my index finger several times to get John to turn around. When he saw the sign, he grimaced, chagrined. I laughed.

"Didn't you wonder where the urinals were?" I asked.

"Well, yeah," John said. "I thought it was kind of strange, but ..."

Back at Mayberry, I parked Pop in the shower room and gave him a haircut. We watched TV with him for awhile, then hugged him and came on home.

I hope you were able to hug your dad today, too, even if only in your heart's memory.

Monday, June 18:

Pop and the social worker

Pop called early this morning. "Barbara, didn't you tell me I didn't have to have a bath today?"

"No, I said you'd need to take one since you didn't on Friday."

"You didn't tell me I didn't have to have a bath?"

"No, Pop. Is Margaret there?"

"Who?"

"Margaret—the lady who helps you with your bath."

"Oh. No, she stuck her head in here a minute ago and told me she'd be back for me in ten minutes." Ah-ha!

"You can't use me for an excuse. Sorry. You need to take one. I'll see you later this morning."

"OK. Bye." he said, disgruntled and abrupt.

Poor man. He'd been hoping for ammunition to fend off Margaret and got no bullets at all. He was sparkling clean by the time Marian, the hospice social worker, arrived. I'm not sure what her purpose is—maybe to give the patient a chance to speak openly about his impending death and his feelings about it—if he wants to. Sometimes families can't deal with and won't talk about it, nor will they allow their loved one to, denying death right up until the last breath is drawn.

Pop greeted Marian with hostility. He didn't know what she could tell him that he didn't already know: He had cancer, it was terminal, his funeral plans were already in place, he could stay at Mayberry until he died, his will was made, John and Barbara loved him, he had a brother and a girlfriend who loved him, he'd made his peace with God and was ready to go when he was called.

Whew! Pop doesn't normally talk at length, so that was quite a speech. Marian smiled and conceded that she really wasn't there to tell him anything. She would just like to visit and get to know him better. She asked what work he'd done before he retired, how long he'd been a widower, and how he'd come to be at Mayberry. Aside from being pretty, she had such a gentle manner that Pop warmed to her considerably.

Forty-five minutes later she told him she'd come back in two weeks, then asked if she could talk with me privately. I walked with her to the front door.

She said Pop would become weaker as the cancer progressed, adding that we might have to hire round-the-clock care when he became too weak to get out of bed; a hospice home-health aide would provide assistance for only an hour a day.

Her comments confused me. I was under the impression that hospice gave more care to patients as the need developed, while family and friends mostly provided emotional and spiritual support. Maybe that's just if you're in a hospice facility? Aside from having a phone number that gives us 24-hour access to a nurse, which gives us access to the doctor and/or pain medication, what do they actually do?

I gotta tell you, I'm concerned about the future, which will most likely involve Pop needing to wear Depends. Mayberry cleans up the residents when they have accidents, but they can't actually pull their adult diapers on and off. (Makes no sense to me, but that's the way it is.)

I'll be spending more time with Pop as he needs increased care, but the man needs to have his dignity. It would mortify him to have me attend to his "personal property." Frankly, I wouldn't be thrilled with that "chore" either. Guess it's time to check the Internet for info.

Sunday, June 24:

Adventures "down home"

Pop's been asking when we were going to have a yard sale at his place. We planned one back in April when it was actually cool, but wet weather interfered. Last month didn't work either because of Pop's isolation, hospitalization, and everything that followed.

Now, just so you know: Anyone who holds a yard sale in Texas between June and September is nuts. It's too darned hot. But Pop probably won't be strong enough for one later this year, so this weekend's gonna have to be it. Since I needed time to get things ready, we decided to go down Wednesday afternoon. John would just have to use more of his vacation hours.

We had some big for-sale items we were going to haul with us in the old clunker truck. Tuesday evening John discovered nails in both its front tires, apparently picked up when he was helping move those cabinets for his church. That meant I could either sit at the tire place for who-knows-how-long Wednesday morning getting them fixed so we could drive the truck and take the big stuff—or I could get the oil changed in the Dodge in ten minutes, drive *it* to Tyler, but leave the big stuff here.

I had a list of ninety-seven things to do without wasting time at the tire place, so it was a two-second decision to leave the big stuff. But the Dodge, which sounded just fine before the oil change, made an air-leaking noise afterwards. God forbid anything should go smoothly.

Well, if I had popped the hood, even I'd have seen the problem, but I didn't. John took a look after he got home. The worker had shown me the air filter, said it was dirty (like I could tell), and did I want him to put in a new one. No. He didn't tighten the cover after he replaced it, so the filter flopped around. Now it was all bent up *and* dirty.

John drove the car back; lifted the hood as the manager walked over, who took one look and said, "Looks like we owe this man an air filter." At least that was easy.

While John took care of that (only ninety-six things left for me to do), I finished loading the Olds, then went to Mayberry to pack up Pop. John arrived, loaded his dad into the Olds; Charlie went into the Dodge with me, and we got on the road.

Even though his porch stairs aren't steep, Pop can't manage them easily anymore. He had to flip his walker up two steps, let it rest against him while he grabbed the railing, pulled himself up those two steps, then flipped the walker again before managing the next two steps. Once at the top, he had to regain his balance before shifting the walker around in order to open the screen and front doors.

He puttered around inside the house for awhile, just glad to be home. Later, John dropped him off at Nancy Lee's so they could visit.

A recent rainstorm had knocked down a tree, almost hitting the house. John worked at clearing away the debris; I stayed inside and did what us "wimmen folk" do—which was methodically go through the house, partly gathering up things for the yard sale, and partly preparing for the carpet cleaners on Thursday. Not only had the carpet not been cleaned in years, but Miss Kitty's former occupancy was still fragrantly apparent.

I got up early Thursday morning because Charlie generally won't let me sleep in. He wanted to go for his walk, dig for gophers and chase rabbits—it was too late (or too early) to howl at the moon. We hadn't gone far when this huge—and I mean *huge*—butterfly landed on a low branch just to my right. I got a good look at it—I swear the wingspan was at least six inches across. When I told John about it, he drawled, "You're in Texas, darlin'—of course it was big. It's a Bubba-fly."

Around 10:30 we got a little worried about Pop since he was still in bed. John finally knocked on his bedroom door and went in. Pop was fine—just enjoying not getting up early. Before moving to Mayberry he used to stay up late watching TV, sleep away the mornings, then microwave a frozen sausage and biscuit sandwich for breakfast. Actually he could still do that at Mayberry if he wanted to, but he won't. I think he thinks he would be a bother if he did.

While John mowed the yard, I started in on the large building that had been both a workshop and storage shed. For some reason I never sifted through it after Mother Pat died—maybe because she died in July and it was too hot in there, or maybe because it was hard enough sorting through her things in the house and in her craft shop.

Mother Pat and Pop are of a generation that never got rid of anything. Didn't matter if it was broken, it was kept because it might be needed. If it was worn out, it was recycled—like the seven-layered sewn-together threadbare washcloth I found.

It's a good thing I love creating order out of chaos because that's what I found in the building—chaos. I maneuvered my way through the clutter to the back wall. Not only had I been smart enough to buy some cool pink leather work gloves to protect my hands, but I also was smart enough to shift things around cautiously, not knowing what might be under or inside. I sure found out fast enough: Furry Critters (mice) and Other Crawling Beasties (BIG bugs—yick.).

As I worked backward toward the door, I moved "keeper" stuff to the rear and everything else to the front. Several hours later I had reaped a small pile of things for the yard sale and a big pile of trash to be hauled off to the dump.

Mark showed up close to noon to take Pop, who was finally up and getting dressed, out to lunch. While he waited, he wanted to help me. I handed things out the door for him to throw into one pile or the other—didn't want him stepping on the wobbly board that served as the stair into the building.

Mark's almost as unsteady on his feet as Pop. He's also blind in one eye, doesn't see that well out of the other, is almost deaf, and his reflexes are slow. Would you ride with this man? Lordy! Lordy!

Pop couldn't get into Mark's full-size truck without John's help, which makes me wonder how he climbed back in after lunch. They drove off.

I was feeling proud of that uncluttered storage building—you could actually walk inside without stepping over anything but the threshold. Then John plunked the chain saw and branch trimmer just inside the doorway, blocking the entrance again. Men!

Mark dropped off Pop just about the time the carpet cleaners were finishing up. He walked toward the house, head and shoulders bent forward. Every few steps he'd stop and "r'are up" to see where he was going. After he passed the craft building, he r'ared up and saw the carpet fellas pulling the hoses back into their truck. He studied them for several seconds before he turned and saw me standing on the porch.

"What in the hell is going on?" he roared, ready to do battle with ne'er-do-wells.

"You just got your carpet cleaned, Pop!" I laughed.

"Oh. Well, OK then." He grinned. "Does it look good?"

"Looks great."

"Good."

Ever since Mother Pat and Pop had the prefab house moved onto their property, the couch served as a dividing line between living room and dining area. Since the cleaners had to move it anyway, I asked them to place it along the wall below the living room window at the front of the house. Doing that not only opened up the space, but now Pop wouldn't have to ease his walker between the couch and a chair to get to his bedroom or the kitchen. Wonder why we never thought of it before.

He seemed pleased with the change. He also commented on the clean carpet before he wandered into his bedroom. John continued cutting tree branches. I decided it was time for a break and took Charlie and my sweaty smelly self off to visit my mom; we went out to eat. I don't know what Pop and John did, but sometimes the men folk just need to fend for themselves. Probably they stalked and snared a couple of wild Whataburgers.

Now a little more history: After moving back to Tyler, Mother Pat bought a small wooden building, had it hauled to their land, set it up right in front of their house, and turned it into her craft shop. She painted and fired greenware of all kinds and made ceramic dolls. She also painted concrete lawn figures which Pop displayed in the yard, near the highway, and sold to passersby.

After she died, he sold almost everything in her estate sale, but quite a few of her creations had been gathering dust in the old shop for the last ten years. When the storage building got too full to get into easily, he started piling things in the shop, too. It's also where John and I had been storing our yard sale stuff from Garland, so it was just as cluttered as the storage building had been.

That is what I had to deal with when John (under protest) and I were up at 6 a.m. Friday. I took Charlie for a short walk while John ate breakfast. Before he left to put up the yard sale signs and to get my mom, he set up three card tables while I spread a couple of tarps on the ground. I started carrying boxes and bags of stuff out of the shop.

John and Mom arrived an hour later. While I continued carting things, already sweaty and tired, John stood in the shade and shopped out of the toolbox Mom wanted to sell. I think I said something rude to him—and strike "think."

Mom had priced her items, but I had neither the time nor inclination to tag ours or Pop's. I just flung numbers at people when they asked. We were hot into sales when Nancy Lee arrived. John took a break from hauling branches down the hill and got Pop out of bed. He and Nancy Lee visited, then she said she'd be back later to take him to Catfish King for supper.

He sat on the porch most of the afternoon, watching the customers, and visiting with whoever had to go inside the house for whatever reason. He told me a couple of times how nice everything looked and how he liked where the couch was, which made me feel good.

Mom is 78 now, overweight, diabetic and severely anemic. She was hot, sunburned and exhausted, even though she'd gone into the house several times to cool off, rest or nap. When we finally closed up late in the afternoon, she tried to help pack up the leftovers, but her face got so red she scared me. I made her go inside.

We sold a lot; it didn't take nearly as long to pack up as it had to unpack—thank goodness. You can actually see the floor in the little shop now. Shortly before I finished, Nancy Lee arrived to take Pop to supper.

We ate microwave dinners, then John took Mom home. After Nancy Lee dropped off Pop, he and John sat on the porch and slapped at the mosquitoes and other flying biting machines. Not my idea of relaxation.

My varicosed legs and bunioned feet were aching from being on them almost constantly for the last three days. I took a shower and went to bed early, just because lying down felt so good.

John later told me that he'd been really annoyed with his dad several times—not because he was sleeping late, but because he mostly seemed to be in another world those three days.

I'm guessing Pop *was* in another world and another time, probably wandering back through memories of his life on that parcel of land. He was born there; he grew up there; given the choice, he'd die there.

He isn't in any hurry to leave us, but I think he's looking forward to "sleeping in." I hope they have a sausage and biscuit breakfast ready for him when he wakes up on the other side.

Wednesday, July 4:

Pop's busy schedule

Last Thursday Pop had an appointment to have his glaucoma pressure checked. I signed him in on a clean sheet so I couldn't see how many other people had signed in for the same time slot. Forty-five minutes later, I walked up to the counter and asked how much longer it would be. Clerk said there were still three people ahead of us—maybe another fifteen minutes. Uh-huh.

Pop, who is usually the Poster Boy of Patience, was disgusted by the long wait, too. Fifteen minutes later we still hadn't been called. He needed to use the restroom, which was in the entry foyer.

We both decided Busy-Doctor didn't need Pop's business. As we passed the sign-in counter, I told the clerk, "Mr. Blanks needs to use the restroom. We won't be back."

She shrugged. She couldn't have cared less.

As we moved across the foyer, Pop watched a woman who was also walking toward the restrooms. He stopped and turned to me. "Did you see how purty that woman is?" When I grinned, he said, irritated, "I'm not so old that I can't appreciate a purty woman."

"I know that, Pop," I said, trying to mollify him.

He felt too tired to attend the Sing Along in the afternoon, but was willing to go to the Open House at John's new church building that evening. We picked him up after supper.

John's church had been located in a shopping-strip store front for several years, but the congregation had increased in numbers, and they desperately needed more space. Last year they got a deal on an old Food Lion building, its parking lot and some surrounding fields. And, yes, the pastor has heard every conceivable joke about Christians and lions since then.

The new Springcreek Church didn't look very "churchy," but you'd never guess it used to be a grocery store either. A construction company did the major remodeling, but volunteers helped finish out the inside. In addition to moving donated cabinets, John dug post holes for the invitational banners, and generally helped where needed. He was our official tour guide at the Open House.

The band was testing the sound system when we arrived and almost blasted us back outside. Apparently making a "joyful noise" equates with making a deafening noise to some people. The volume was physically painful for me, and I put my fingers in my ears. John has some hearing loss, but said it was too loud for him. Even Pop turned off his hearing aids.

As we wandered back to the area where several classrooms were, John pointed out the stairs leading to the "attic." He said a burglar had broken in through the roof last week, not realizing he'd set off a silent alarm. When the cops arrived, they didn't know the floor plan of the new church, so they let the police dogs loose.

The dogs quickly found the man, and the cops found them by following the man's screams and the trail of his blood. He was trying to exit out the same hole he'd entered through, but the dogs had their jaws clamped to his anatomy.

"Well, dog *is* God spelled backwards," I said, "which just proves if you break into His house, God will bite your butt."

After we took the tour, Pop helped to break in the new men's room—an entirely different wag of the tail, so to speak.

Yesterday Marian, the hospice social worker, visited again. She told me afterwards that Pop had been hostile when she called; he didn't understand why she was coming to see him. "Anything you want to know you can talk to Barbara or John about." She told him it was routine and went anyway.

She arrived a half hour earlier than she'd predicted, so I didn't witness her un-welcome, but her personality is such that she charmed him. In fact, he had enjoyed telling stories about his oil field days, his farming life and his limited war experiences to a pretty lady.

And then Lori, the hospice RN, came to see Pop today (despite it being a holiday) because she was going on vacation and wanted to check on him before she left. John hadn't met her yet, so we made it a point to be at Mayberry before she arrived.

Pop hadn't eaten lunch—he said his stomach hurt. That gave me a little flutter of fear: "Oh no, it's starting ..." The pain was gone by the time Lori examined him though. He told her he hadn't been sleeping well because of intense itching that moved from his arms to his back to his legs to all over. Lori suggested he take two Tylenol PM with his evening meds. The antihistamine in it is both itch reliever and sleep-aid.

When she finished her exam, Pop joked, "Will I live till I die?" Lori laughed.

After she left, he and John decided to drive around for awhile. They picked me up later, and we drove directly to Braum's. By then Pop was hungry. I put my arm around Pop's shoulder as we walked inside—it was scary how bony he felt. And how could I possibly be as tall as he was now? Had he shrunk that much?

He spoiled his appetite for supper by ordering a hamburger, fries and a chocolate shake. Ate most of it, too.

Monday, July 9:

Pop and John

Pop had a "routine visit" with the oncologist this morning. He showed a black, scabby thing on his chest to Dr. O, who said he could scrape it off for biopsy—or we could have his primary physician do it. We hadn't seen Dr. A since the hepatitis fiasco and decided to take it to him. Well, mostly I decided.

Other than that, Pop's doing well enough that the oncologist actually seemed bored with him. Hey, that's a good thing!

Some of you have been asking how John's been doing. He has his good and bad moments.

Although it doesn't matter to the story what the baggage is, John has a love/dislike ("hate" is too strong) relationship with his dad. Even though he's being forced to deal with those conflicting emotions, the love he feels for his dad far outstrips anything else. He's already grieving.

Tonight he cried—hard. His daddy is dying.

Thursday, July 12:

Getting personal

I'm telling you this because you may have a man in your life who could use this product. We knew it was made for women—at least it was associated in my mind that way—but there are also absorbent pads designed specifically for men who can't hold their bladders.

Yesterday, when Pop complained about his problem to Lori, she told us about them. After she left, I went shopping. Sure enough— Depends for Men. I bought a package and went back to Mayberry. I pulled out a pad and showed it to Pop, saying John could show him how to put it on later.

He eyed it, then picked his words carefully. "That's kind of like the Kotex ladies wear, isn't it?"

Oh dear! I tried hard not to laugh because that's exactly what I'd thought. I placed my hand on his shoulder while I ducked my head and tried to think what to say.

"Well, kind of like that, Pop, but these are made especially for men...in case you can't get to the bathroom in time."

He stared at nothing for several seconds, an odd little smile on his face. Finally he said he didn't really think he needed them, but he'd have John show him what to do.

Today we kept our appointment with Dr. A, even though Pop told me this morning that the sore on his chest was almost gone. I began to suspect the crusty thing might have been a scab covering a big pimple.

When Dr. A entered the exam room, I noticed his hair style was different—spiky, like he'd just towel-dried it but hadn't combed it. When I commented, he sheepishly admitted his wife had grown tired of his Dr. Kildare-look and had sent him to her stylist. I just shook my head, grinning at him. We moved on.

"We're probably here on a false alarm," I said.

He looked at the wound. Yep, the scab covered a healing pimple, although he said some basal cell cancers start out looking like that. He gave Pop a brief exam, but mostly he just talked with us. I think he appreciated that we'd come in.

Before we left, Pop made Dr. A chuckle by saying, "I guess I'm gonna to live till I die." That's his favorite line now.

Monday, July 16:

The chaplain's chat

Pop wanted a haircut before Janet, the hospice chaplain, came for the first time. He was sitting on the porch in spite of the heat, so we had our barber session out there. I'd finally been smart enough to get an extension cord for the razor, so we didn't block the front door. For someone mostly bald, that man grows a lot of hair.

Janet showed up—late. She was nice enough, but she didn't seem to be much at ease. Pop was a little uneasy, too—probably because he didn't know what she expected from him. She tried to draw him out, but he didn't respond to her the way he did to the social worker.

Actually, Janet did most of the talking herself, then asked if she could say a prayer. Pop allowed as how he was always ready for a prayer, whipped off his glasses, covered his eyes, and let her commence…and commence…and commence.

After she left, I asked him, "Well, what did you think?"

"Long winded, isn't she."

Cracked me up. He'd only said what I'd been thinking. He appreciated her effort, but he hoped I'd be there the next time she came —meaning, "please don't leave me alone with her."

John just talked with Pop, who's decided he really doesn't want to talk with Janet again—nor does he want to talk to any ministers; he doesn't need one because he already talks directly to the Lord.

Thursday, July 19:

Ups and downs

Pop's been having stomach pain more frequently these last couple of weeks, but he felt well enough Monday night to let us know he'd run out of his Little Debbie brownies.

I took him a box on Tuesday. He was slumped in his chair, rubbing his stomach. When he saw me, he said, "I feel bloated." To prove it, he pressed on his belly and belched, making me snort through my nose, which made him repeat the performance several times until we were both laughing.

Moments later his eyes looked sad. He said, "I'm feeling pretty blue, Barbara, but I reckon I'll feel perkier once my belly quits hurting so much."

The bloat isn't funny—it means the cancer has grown to where it's really starting to affect him. Maybe I should have let it go, but we have been honest with him from the first. Sometimes I hate that. I told him that the pain and bloating were symptoms of the pancreatic cancer, and they weren't going to go away. (I didn't realize until I verbalized it to him that I had been thinking they would go away, too. Damn, damn, damn.)

"I'm not scared to die," he said, but then he started crying. He kept slapping his knee, saying, "I wish I'd just hurry up and get it over with." He apologized for talking about his troubles.

"Pop, you can always talk to me or John. Listen, your feelings are your feelings. You shouldn't apologize for them." He repeated that a couple of times, as if to reassure himself. Then he asked how long it was until the next memorial service at the cemetery in Tyler.

"It's a month away."

"I really would like to go to one more memorial. Do you think I can make it till then, Barbara?"

"I don't know, Pop. I sure hope so."

I called Lori the nurse then. She said she'd prefer he stay on Tylenol as long as possible, since all the other painkillers would cause drowsiness; Gas-X would help relieve the bloat.

As I was getting ready to leave, I asked Pop to give me one more toot for the road. He grinned, pressed his stomach and belched. Gabriella knocked then and asked if she could come in to clean his bathroom. That's when he thought to tell me Margaret was sick, so he hadn't had a bath on Monday. Gabriella said she could give him one on Wednesday, and kidded him—it wouldn't be like a stranger was bathing him, and he'd be covered with a towel anyway.

"How about giving him a bath right now?" I said.

"I could do that," she said, playing along.

"Whoa!" Pop bellowed, almost falling out of his chair. Gabriella and I laughed. I thought it best to leave before Pop threw me out.

Yesterday he told me he had talked Gabriella out of his bath by telling her she could bathe him on Friday instead. He looked sideways at me and gave me that sly grin of his.

"We're going to Tyler on Friday, aren't we?"

"Uh-uh, we're going Saturday."

"Dang!" he said, shaking his head. "I messed up. I should have told her she could give me my bath on Saturday."

I couldn't help laughing. Poor Pop—too cunning for his own bad memory.

Two weeks ago, after we'd walked out on that ophthalmologist, I'd called a mobile eye-doctor. Today was exam day, and I high-tailed it to Mayberry. Pop was sitting on the porch next to Miss Dorothy, who is a sweet, soft-spoken lady. He's commented a couple of times how much he enjoys talking with her and how pretty she is.

I had just finished telling him the optometrist would arrive soon, when the van pulled up. When Pop realized he had to go inside, he got mad, grousing that he wanted to continue his conversation with Dorothy. He did *not* appreciate the interruption. But he stood up and stalked inside.

Miss Dorothy retreated to her room. A short time later she came back out and passed through the dining room where Pop was being examined. I watched him as he watched her. His eyes moved from her head down to her legs and back up again—several times.

They really never get too old to look, do they?

The doctor spent over a half-hour with Pop—personalized care at its best. His glaucoma pressure tested fine, and his general eye exam indicated his vision is good for his age. It's certainly still good enough to appreciate the female form.

I debated whether I should tell you this or not, but you might as well know the rest of it. Maybe it seems—well—dumb for Pop to have an eye exam when he has only a few months left. But it never occurred to me to not have his eyes checked.

While the doctor examined him, his assistant and I sat at a dining table and talked. At some point, I'm ashamed to say, I smarted off and said, "We don't want Pop to go blind before he dies." As the words came out, my eyes filled with tears. I hadn't realized they were so close to the surface. Sometimes the reality of his cancer is more real than at other times. This totally sucks.

Monday, July 23:

Pop gets cranky

When we went to Tyler on Saturday, I spent the day with my mom. John almost got heat stroke from cutting grass with the old push lawn mower because he couldn't start the riding mower. Pop wandered around his house or sat on the porch. He wouldn't go see his girlfriend or his brother—wouldn't say why; he just didn't want to go.

Today I hit Walmart for more Tylenol, Gas-X and birdseed. When I saw Pop after lunch, it struck me again that he is visibly thinner; his face especially is looking skeletal.

Several of the ladies were still sitting around one of the dining tables. Miss Bess, with her Lucille Ball henna-red hair, had been in Mississippi with her daughter last week. I gave her a welcome-back hug before she went out on the porch to have a cigarette.

Kellie offered me the last piece of chocolate pie from lunch. "Anyone want to share this with me?" I asked. Miss Frances and Miss Clara did. I grabbed three forks, cut the slice into three slivers, and set the pie plate in the middle of the table—no point in dirtying dishes. We were down to the last bite when Miss Bess came back in, grabbed a fork, and finished it off.

Miss Frances sat back in her chair. She's always bundled up in warm clothes even though the thermostat is set too high for us young'uns. She's too old to do anything but speak her mind, so when she noticed my running shoes, she said, "Those are really ugly shoes."

"I know," I said, laughing, "but they don't hurt my feet. They're expensive, too, because they charge extra for ugly."

"They must have cost a fortune," she wisecracked.

I got Pop's meds box from the locked "safe room" and brought it to the table to add the Tylenol and Gas-X. Miss Clara, who has more energy than most of the other ladies but is developing Alzheimer's, jabbered away to no one in particular. I really wasn't paying attention—until Pop leaned over to me and quietly growled, "That's the kind of *crap* I have to put up with every day."

Miss Clara heard. She turned on him.

"What did you say?"

"What makes you think I was talking to you?" Pop snapped, his annoyance with her out in the open.

I glanced at Kellie who was cleaning off the other table; she didn't look at me or say anything. I ducked my head and prepared to slide under the table if necessary.

Miss Clara demanded to know what Pop had said. He repeated it. She flared something at him.

I imitated a turtle, pulling my head down into my hunched shoulders, trying to make myself invisible. One more back-and-forth, then Clara stormed off. Pop wasn't the least bit sorry.

Where's Sheriff Andy Taylor when you need him? He was always real good at smoothing things over.

Thursday, July 26:

Pop sings along

When we put our brains together, Kellie and I are pretty smart. Pop has been taking Pancrease capsules to help his body absorb nutrients. The prescription said take three with each meal. When his appetite decreased, I reduced the number to two, thinking he didn't need three when he didn't have much food in his stomach. Then I started worrying that maybe it was hurting him to not get the full dose, and I raised it back to three.

Well, Kellie sometimes called me to question it, because she noticed when he ate little and took three capsules, his stomach would hurt later, but he was OK if he took three after a larger meal. We decided we'd better check that out.

I called hospice, and was told Pancrease should be given proportional to food intake because it's a "mucosal irritant." Jeez, why isn't it written up that way in the instructions?

This afternoon Pop felt so good he was already in the audience for the Sing Along with Winona by the time I arrived. As she played "5 Foot 2, Eyes of Blue," I could hear him singing under his breath, "but oh what those five foot could do ..." (He must have been thinking about Mother Pat. She was actually 5'1" but told everyone she was 5'2" because she wanted to be taller.)

Pop started out sporting a star-spangled top hat, then Winona swapped it for that engineer's cap he wore at our first Sing Along. When we started singing "I've Been Working on the Railroad," I leaned near his ear and prompted, "Say Toot Toot!" He did! Every time I said, "Toot Toot," Pop grinned and sang it out.

During the next song, Winona encouraged everyone to "Shake your maracas!"

"Shake it but don't break it—it's already cracked," Pop mouthed quietly.

He was definitely feeling nostalgic. When John was eleven, he and his folks were visiting relatives in Louisiana. One evening everyone went out for dinner at a "beer joint"—back when they were family diners as well as places of entertainment. Pop had a few beers—John said it was the first time he'd ever seen his dad drink. He was feeling good by the time the show started, so when the "wiggle dancer" came on, Pop shouted, "Shake it but don't break it—it's already cracked." It certainly made an impression on John.

Anyway, Pop not only "heckled" Winona into dancing the Charleston, but he also spoke up at the end of the show and said everyone should give her a round of applause. We did.

While she played "Boogie Woogie Bugle Boy" on her flute, I gathered up the props she'd distributed—song sheets, hats, flags, and the maracas—which I shook along my booty. Everyone clapped, laughed and enjoyed seeing me be silly. Pop had such a good time he told John all about it later.

Friday, July 27:

Pop is not doing well

Kellie called me at work today—right after Pop threw up three times while sitting at the lunch table. I asked her to call the hospice nurse, quickly finished up the job I was doing, then left for Mayberry.

By the time I arrived, just an hour after Kellie's call, Pop had become jaundiced, had tremors in his arms, couldn't walk, and his temperature fluctuated between chills and fever. A dramatic change from yesterday—obviously. He says he's not in pain, which is good, especially since we've been told pancreatic cancer can become excruciatingly painful as the tumor grows and presses against other organs.

Valerie, a hospice nurse, arrived, checked his vitals, and noted his heartbeat was irregular. She decided to put him on continuous-care over the weekend so he could be fully evaluated. That meant LVNs would be with him on twelve-hour shifts.

I asked her why he was jaundiced—the metal stent was supposed to prevent it. She said it could be occluded—overgrown— by the cancer growth, which is apparently what has happened.

Valerie asked Pop some questions—testing for stroke, I think. She asked what day it was. He thought it was Tuesday—wasn't sure—but he often loses track of the days. He knew who he was, where he was, who I was. No problem there. She asked if he knew who the president is.

"Why sure. George Bush."

Then she asked something she shouldn't have: "Did you vote for him?" Pop hesitated. I started laughing.

"Barbara ..." he said in an exasperated, "darn you" tone. He shook his head and smiled his "you caught me" grin, then looked directly at Valerie.

"No, I did not," he stated emphatically.

Guess that told her.

Saturday, July 28:

Pop is a little better today

We half-expected he would die last night, he was that bad. This morning, when Charlie and I walked over to Mayberry, he seemed better—still yellow, but no tremors, no fever, no vomiting.

The nurse had just helped him lie down for a nap after breakfast. She sorta tried to stop us from going into his room, so we just sorta breezed right by her. Pop was lying on his side with his back to the door. We walked around to his front. He hadn't even dozed off yet.

"I brought someone to see you, Pop." I patted the bed. Charlie leaped up, waggled everything, and gave him doggy kisses.

"You rascal!" Pop laughed and patted him. His voice sounded stronger. It always perks him up to see Charlie. We talked a minute before the nurse said she was going to get Pop into a wheelchair later and take him down the hall for a bath.

"Didn't I have a bath yesterday?" he protested. Yep, his voice was definitely stronger.

"Yes, but trust me—you need another one," I said. "I bet you can't talk your way out of it either like you do with Margaret." He scowled but didn't say anything.

Charlie and I didn't stay long. Pop really was tired.

Sunday, July 29:

Pop is very weak

He mostly sleeps now. His stomach feels sore when he presses on it, so of course John and I tell him to quit pressing. Still, he says he's not in any real pain. I'm not sure if he's saying that to ease our minds or if it's true.

But it does ease our minds to know that at some point Pop stopped being afraid of dying. He didn't actually say the words, but something in his demeanor changed. Acceptance? Peace? I don't know, but he isn't afraid.

+++++

A hospice nurse-manager met us at Mayberry this evening to evaluate Pop. His body shows some signs of shutting down, but not enough to warrant keeping him on continuous care. Instead, "custodial care" will begin tomorrow evening—meaning an hour-a-day aide will come in to give bed baths and other personal assistance—I'm not exactly sure what that entails.

But he definitely needs help. He can't sit up or walk by himself —he's essentially become as weak and as helpless as a baby. His life has come full circle.

John and I visited three nursing homes in Garland this afternoon. I'm surprised I was coherent enough to ask questions since I woke up at 4:30 this morning with Pop on my mind and couldn't go back to sleep.

The first nursing home stunk—looked clean but it stunk. The director tried to pass it off as lunchtime food smells, but ain't *no* way it was food. At least, I hope it wasn't. The other two places didn't smell —as much—but they had fewer nurses and aides per patients/residents than the first place. All three were horribly depressing. We've definitely been spoiled by the homey atmosphere of Mayberry.

After leaving the third place, we agreed that I would start calling home-care agencies on Monday. We picked up Charlie, then went to see Pop. We offered to get him a Whataburger and chocolate milk shake, but he said, "Maybe tomorrow." His voice was weak again, and the tremors in his arms were back.

He asked John about the cemetery memorial service in Whitehouse, repeating his desire to go. John tried to sound upbeat about it, assuring his dad by half-teasing, "You'll make it there one way or the other, Pop." But he took Charlie outside immediately after that. When they returned, John's eyes were red.

While they were gone, I sat at Pop's left side and lightly stroked his chest. He looked me in the eyes.

"Barbara, I want you to tell me the truth. Do you think I'll be able to go to the memorial?"

Honesty be damned—I just couldn't just give him a flat "No."

"I don't know," I hedged. "You'd have to be strong enough to make the drive, and you'd have to be strong enough to climb your porch stairs. If you aren't strong enough, then no, you couldn't go."

Bless him, he didn't ask me if I thought he'd be strong enough.

Before we went home again, John helped Pop sit up so he could use the urinal bottle. I retreated to the kitchen where Cortney had just taken pans of cupcakes out of the oven.

We compared bleary eyes—she hadn't slept well last night either from thinking about Pop. After a couple of minutes I realized I was drooling. "When are you going to frost those cupcakes—hint hint?"

"I guess I can frost one right now." She did, and as she handed it to me, she started crying. "I get so attached to them and then they die."

I set the cupcake on the counter, and held her while she sobbed into my shoulder. She's one of the reasons we want Pop to stay at Mayberry.

Monday, July 30:

Pop is failing

John and I just got back from taking Charlie to the emergency clinic. He'll be OK, but we sure didn't need another crisis.

Pop had been stable when we left him last night, but deteriorated rapidly after that. He was so bad that his regular hospice nurse, Lori, re-evaluated him this morning. She saw several indications that he is almost ready to leave us. She consulted with her boss, and based on his condition now, they are keeping him on continuous care. They think his condition is "imminent."

That means he probably has forty-eight to seventy-two hours left.

That's all I feel up to telling you tonight.

Tuesday morning, July 31:

It will be very soon

Pop is essentially non-responsive today.

His brother and nephew came to see him. Mark's taking it real hard. John's pastor and assistant pastor also came and prayed over Pop. I made it clear to the hospice nurse that we wanted an open door policy so the ladies could come in to see him. Kellie, his house angel, comes in as often as she can; she cries right along with us.

I'm going to start gathering and packing for Whitehouse in a minute. Maybe that sounds a little cold, but it's just easier to be busy and to handle practicalities.

So many of you care about Pop—I can't begin to tell you how much that means to me. I'll try to keep you updated as much as possible.

Tuesday evening, July 31:

Pop hasn't left yet

It's almost 10 p.m. Central. Pop isn't quite ready to leave yet. He's still non-responsive, except twice his facial expression changed when—

I'm sorry. I'll have to tell you later. It's too hard right now.

Pop had a busy day what with his brother, nephew, two pastors, and several ladies visiting him. He looks comfortable, but if he moans or seems to be hurting, the nurse gives him—morphine sulfate, I think, sublingually.

She will call us if his condition worsens during the night.

So many of you have sent me personal notes, and while I still haven't had a chance to read them, I appreciate that you wrote and will get back to you later.

Pop will probably leave us tomorrow.

Wednesday, August 1:

Pop is gone

He died at 11:35 p.m. Tuesday night. He left quietly and easily.

169

John and I had just gone to bed when the call came. Pop had had a full day and was real tired. He was glad—on some level—for all the company, but he didn't want to be rude and die while he had visitors.

We said our good-byes to him while we waited for the hospice RN nurse to arrive to pronounce him (the LVN couldn't do it), and then for the mortuary service to pick him up. Pop is going home to stay.

It's almost 3:30 a.m. now, but I wanted you to know.

Saturday, August 4:

We're back

I'll tell you about Pop's last two days and the aftermath soon.

Several cards from ya'll were waiting for us, but I haven't had a chance to open them yet. Thank you for now though.

John and I are exhausted.

Sunday, August 5:

Pop…easing into the rest of his story

So many of you have shared in Pop's life for the last fifteen months. You've said he reminds you of your own dad or father-in-law or husband. One woman told me her kids "adopted" him as their grandpa. You've told me stories about someone you love who's going through or went through something similar, and how his stories have helped you to reconcile your losses. You've cared about him, and that's why it feels right to tell you the rest.

As strange as it sounds, in spite of knowing he had pancreatic cancer, in spite of all the evidence of his approaching death, in spite of preparing for it, I still never *really* expected Pop to die. Anyway, I'm going to recap a little here, partly for my sake, but also to fill y'all in on some things I hadn't been able to tell you before.

Pop joined the lunch group on Friday the 27th, although he had pretty much quit eating and drinking anything by then. You wouldn't think he'd have much to vomit, but he managed to do a good job of it. Shortly after he grossed out everyone, he developed jaundice, muscle tremors, and rapid temperature fluctuations. (The body's thermostat goes haywire as the bile toxins build up in the brain.)

We looked at nursing homes on Sunday because we thought hospice continuous-care would end soon. Late that same night Dianne called John and asked him to come help Pop off the commode. He couldn't get himself up, and the LVN and Dianne together couldn't lift him. Then she thought of Michael—he and his wife are managers of House 1. She'd try to get hold of him first. John and I dozed off again without hearing anything further from her.

John went to work as usual Monday morning. Before I began the private nursing care search, I called the day-LVN to check on Pop. She said he'd had a bad night—bad enough that Lori, his regular hospice RN, would be re-evaluating him later that morning.

The nurse asked if we had told him it was "OK" for him to leave us. Yes, sort of. We had paraphrased Pop's own words and told him that we were ready to let him go when he was ready to go, but we weren't in any hurry about it.

Her question alarmed me though. "Is he really that bad?"

"Yes, he is."

I called John, who let his boss know the current situation, then headed home.

As he aged, Pop became afraid—afraid of doing something wrong, afraid of bothering us, afraid he already was or would become a burden. It didn't matter how many times we assured him otherwise, he worried about it. Ever since he moved into Mayberry he'd been telling us, "I'm trying to be good. I'm trying to do everything I'm supposed to."

Suddenly I knew the right thing to say. When John arrived, I repeated what the LVN had said. Then I said, "I think I know what we need to tell your dad: You've been good, Pop. You've done everything you were supposed to do. It's OK if you want to leave now."

John whirled away, slammed his hand against the wall, and started crying. When he could speak again, he thanked me. He, too, thought it was exactly what his dad needed hear.

I need to take a break here. This is hard.

Tuesday, August 7:

Pop's last two days

So John and I went to Mayberry together. The nurse hadn't exaggerated—Pop's condition had deteriorated drastically. The jaundice had deepened from yellow to "orange as a pumpkin." His arms moved restlessly, and his fingers kept picking at the sheet. His eyelids were half-closed, but his eyes constantly flicked back and forth.

He could speak, but between not wearing his dentures, not moving his lips, and his dry mouth, he sounded like someone talking through dental cotton. When we couldn't understand him, he became agitated. Sometimes he spoke to people who weren't there—well, to people we couldn't see anyway.

When Pop was first diagnosed, hospice wanted to switch him to a hospital bed. He adamantly refused to allow it. However, he was so weak that Lori thought it was time; she would order delivery of one for later that day. We hadn't realized he was listening until he spoke up.

"Don't be in such an all-fired hurry to get rid of my bed!" he said. We sure understood him that time. Unfortunately, it had to be done.

After Lori observed Pop and checked his physical signs, she determined he was no longer "custodial" but "imminent," meaning she expected he would die within forty-eight to seventy-two hours. She consulted with her supervisors, and they agreed to keep him on continuous care.

We asked Lori to speak plainly to us about what to expect, so she outlined the progression the body takes as it shuts down. One of the first signs is refusing food and drink. The restlessness and picking at the sheet are other signs. The LVNs reported him passing "small gray stools," another sign of approaching death. Lori said Pop would soon reach a state of non-responsiveness to everything except hearing.

"That's the last thing to go."

I actually laughed. "Pop's hearing was the first thing to go years ago—we'd better make sure he's wearing his hearing aids so he can hear us at the last."

John went back to work just long enough to update his boss and to tie up a few loose ends. I stayed with Pop, sitting on the bed at his left side because he kept his head turned that way. I frequently

172

patted his chest or stroked his arm; I'm not certain if I was trying to comfort him or me—probably me.

I am tremendously grateful to hospice for all they did, and Pop liked having the nurses fuss over him, but I wanted to strangle the one I think of as Clarabelle —like the clown—but she wasn't funny. I keep blocking on her real name.

Even when my back was to her, Clarabelle responded as if I was talking to her—thus drowning out anything Pop said. Or she rattled her paperwork so loudly when he spoke that I couldn't hear him. She also exhaled these huge "I'm overworked and under-appreciated" SIGHs. Sometimes I could barely manage *not* to scream, "SHUT UP!" at her.

She kept removing Pop's hearing aids—even knowing he could still hear us but couldn't hear without them. And she wouldn't let the ladies into his room—even after I explicitly told her they could visit him. He considered them family. She had no right to keep them out.

Thank goodness she sometimes left the room. It was during one of her absences that I told Pop, "You're the best Pop in the whole world." His eyebrows shot upwards and his eyes opened wide.

"Weelwee?" Unable to speak clearly, but said so earnestly he made me cry.

"Yes, really. I wouldn't lie to you. You're the best Pop in the whole world." He smiled a proud, pleased, toothless smile.

+++++

John came directly to Mayberry after he finished up at work; I had to go home for awhile. Maybe it sounds awful, but I grabbed an armful of clothes from Pop's closet and took them with me. After that I almost always carried something out of his room. My practical side was trying to make things easier for us later.

At home, I called Nancy Lee to update her on Pop's condition, paid attention to Charlie, then returned to Mayberry. The hospital bed had just been delivered and was being set up. Pop had been moved to the wheelchair, but his bones had dissolved. It took both John and me to keep him from sliding to the floor.

Michael from House 1 came over about that time. He and John shifted Pop onto the new bed, then carried the old bed out to our truck. Clarabelle got him settled, and gave him a pain killer because he was moaning. He wanted to rest.

John and I left, returning after we ate supper. John stood at the head of the bed while I reclaimed Pop's left side. When John spoke, Pop lurched and cried out, trying to turn his head toward the source of the booming voice.

"Who's that?"

"It's me, Pop—John."

"*Who?*"

"Move around to where he can see you," I suggested. Pop visibly relaxed when he saw John. I laughed and said that reminded me of the show where Archie Bunker was trapped in his basement, got drunk, heard a deep, authoritative voice speaking from the top of the basement stairs, and thought it was God.

Since Pop was stable, I went home, which is when I discovered Charlie was having a problem and needed to go to the emergency clinic. I called John. He told his dad he had to leave and why.

In the first show of strength he'd had all day, he asked, "Who's going with you?"

John: "Barbara is."

Pop, trying to get up: "I'm going with you!"

John, placing his hand on Pop's chest: "You can't go with me— you're not strong enough."

Pop, shouting: "You *watch* me! Get my boots! I'll *show* you!"

He started struggling. He kicked Clarabelle in the stomach. (Honestly, it pleased me to hear that.)

"*Give me my gun!*" he yelled. "I'll *shoot* you!"

It was all John and Clarabelle could do to keep him in bed until Debra, the night shift LVN who had just arrived, could give him a sedative.

That incident used up the last of his strength. His condition went from responsive to non-responsive overnight. He lay unmoving; even his eyes were still behind his barely-open eyelids. He never spoke again.

Lori arrived Tuesday morning, a little surprised, I think, to find him failing so rapidly. "Imminent" became from twenty-four to forty-eight hours. What "imminent" really means is someone is counting down the clock, then ready or not, there you go.

After she left, I told Pop, "I called Nancy Lee…" As soon as I said her name, his eyebrows rose in an attitude of listening. It lasted only a moment, but it was the first time his expression had changed since he'd become non-responsive.

It made me sad that Mark couldn't see Pop on Monday when they still could have talked. But he can't make the long drive by himself, and Mark, Jr. couldn't bring him sooner. When they came into the room on Tuesday, Clarabelle wouldn't get out of their way. She kept rubbing Pop's chest, calling him "darlin'," messing with his blankets—putting on a show for the newcomers. (Where's your gun, Pop?)

Somehow John forced her aside so Mark could sit near his brother. He talked to him, cried, and squeezed "Johnny's" hand—he felt sure Johnny squeezed back. After awhile Mark, Jr. and John helped him walk to the back porch so he could collect himself.

I let them know when Pastor Keith and Associate Pastor Susan arrived to pray over Pop. With six of us crowded around the bed, Clarabelle finally took the hint and left the room. At some point I was standing next to Keith when he asked me if I was all right. "No," I squeaked, and started crying. He put his arm around my shoulders, which only made me cry more.

Keith and Susan left, then Mark and Mark, Jr. John went home for awhile—to ride the exercise bike. He hadn't moved around much for two days, and it was a good way to relieve some of his tension. Kellie had fixed Hobo Stew for lunch, and when she offered me a bowl, I sat in Pop's chair at the table and ate with the ladies.

After lunch, when we were alone in his room, I once again told him, "You're the best Pop in the whole world."

Instantly his eyebrows shot upwards, his almost-closed eyes opened a little wider, his jaw dropped in an expression of complete surprise...and then his whole face collapsed into the most beautiful, pleased, proud, face scrunched-up smile I've ever seen. He absolutely beamed.

And, yes, I cried. A moment later his face became passive again. That was the last time he responded to anything.

When Miss Bess and Kellie came to his door, I very pointedly looked at Clarabelle and announced we were having an Open Door policy all day. Even then—even *then* she tried to keep people out—and with me standing there. I overrode her several times—too bad I didn't have a tank to do it with. Miss Margaret would have bull-dozed her way in if she'd been there, but she was in the hospital having surgery for colon cancer. Dianne was with her mother, of course.

175

Michael came over several times and just stood at Pop's bedside. He and Pop used to sit on the porch in the evenings and talk about hunting, fishing, farming and other things—like raising chickens. Pop had mentioned him to me a few times—that he enjoyed talking with a young man—but never mentioned Michael by name. Probably couldn't remember it.

John and I stayed until Debra, the night-LVN arrived. Pop was comfortable and unchanged. Lori had told us advanced indications of approaching death would be a spiking temperature (like a radiator overheating) and the non-breathing moments would become longer than the breathing moments. Pop's temperature hadn't come close to spiking, and his breathing was rapid but normal. We all thought it would be "safe" for us to go home for the night.

But Yvette, the night-shift lady for House 2, called us just before midnight.

"You'd better come."

John and I hurriedly threw on some clothes and raced that long, long one mile to Mayberry. We rushed inside, thinking Pop was still alive. Debra told us, "He's gone," as we flew past her and into his room; it didn't register with me.

As we stood on opposite sides of his bed, I waited for his next breath, thinking Pop was in that breathing/not-breathing stage. The moment realization struck, I felt this wail rising up in my chest, and clapped my hand over my mouth to muffle the sound. John came around the bed, and held me. Then he broke down, too.

That was the hardest moment. All these years we had slowed down to wait for Pop, to move at his pace, and then he couldn't wait for us.

Debra respected our privacy. She waited until she heard nose-blowing before she came in. She said about ten minutes after she'd last checked Pop's vital signs, she heard him take a breath, waited for the next one—and it never came. She glanced at the clock as she went to his side. It was 11:35 p.m., Tuesday, July 31.

An LVN can't legally pronounce a death, so Debra called Marlene, a hospice RN who lives in Garland. Marlene pronounced at 1 a.m., August 1, so that is the legal time and date on the death certificate.

While we were waiting for her, John called the funeral home in Tyler, which contacted the mortuary service in Dallas, which arrived about forty-five minutes later. He also went next door to tell Michael,

176

who came and stood by Pop for several minutes, before going out to the dining room; he slumped into a chair.

Yvette made coffee, bless her. After the mortuary man arrived, Marlene, Debra, and I stood at the kitchen counter and talked. Actually, mostly I talked, telling them stories about Pop—it was like I knew if my mouth stopped moving, I'd collapse.

I also told Debra I was glad that she was with him when he died, not Clarabelle, and explained why. She appreciated knowing that.

It seemed like John and the mortuary man were in Pop's room for a long time. I never asked John for details. All I know is he helped move him from bed to gurney, then covered his body with a red, plush shroud. He said it was the last thing he could do for his dad.

Pop was always the gentleman. He waited until all the ladies were asleep so they wouldn't have to watch while the mortuary man, John and Michael rolled him away.

He didn't bother anyone.

Marlene and Debra left. John got Pop's suit out of his closet, we took a look around, then left his room. I don't know why, but as I closed the door, I quoted, "So long, and thanks for all the fish." John choked out a laugh. He understood the reference, but for those who haven't read Douglas Adams' book—that's the parting line of the dolphins as they are leaving the earth, just before it's destroyed.

John got to bed about 3:30 a.m. I stayed up to let y'all know about Pop.

Charlie seemed depressed—he'd been left alone too much lately
—so I grabbed a pillow and curled up on the floor next to him. He finally sighed, relaxed and slept, as did I.

We were up again at seven. We finished packing, got the cars loaded; we each made several phone calls. We managed to leave for Tyler about 10:30, never thinking to take Pop's underwear or shoes or a picture of him.

Wednesday, August 8:

The aftermath

When we reached Pop's place, we found Mark sitting on the front porch steps. John and I sat down on either side of him, and we cried together.

After that, we unloaded the car and got Charlie settled. We had to take Pop's suit to the funeral home, and tried to get Mark to go with us, but he decided to return to Longview.

Pop and Mother Pat had bought pre-arranged, full-service funerals a few years before she died. Because of their advance planning, we essentially just had to decide how many death certificates to order and fill out the form for the newspaper obituary. John signed paperwork "canceling" the full-service contract, replacing it with instructions for a graveside service only, because that's what Pop had said he wanted now.

John choked up several times and couldn't talk; I was OK—dealing with practicalities, you see. Then Steve, the funeral man, left to type up the info. John left to use the restroom. I sat in the office by myself and cried.

John signed the typed papers. Steve said they'd provide the underwear and shoes we forgot to bring. He showed us a silver-grey coffin, a twin to Mother Pat's. It was a work of art with its long, sleek lines and beautiful creamy-white smocked lining—seemed a shame to bury something that lovely.

Done there, we walked across the street to order a spray of flowers for the casket. After that we picked up my mom (who stayed with us for the duration), ate an early supper, and went back to Pop's. Nancy Lee came over, bringing a cake, and we told her about the last two days.

We returned to the funeral home Thursday morning to "approve" Pop's appearance. He didn't look like he was asleep. He didn't look "natural." He looked "fine" though. He'd also had a manicure—his nails looked like he'd never worked a day in his life. I wonder if they tried to trim his thick, tough toenails—makes me smile to think about it.

I don't want to gross out anybody, but here's what puzzles me. A funeral home keeps a body in cold storage whether it's embalmed or not, so the coldness of it I understand. Why, though, does a body feel so *heavy* when you touch it—not to lift any part of it, but just the feel of it, even through a suit jacket?

Maybe a person's "buoyancy" comes from breathing, from the air in the body tissues. I suppose some people think it comes from the soul, and when that's gone, only a concrete-heavy lump of flesh is left. I don't know. I just know that heavy feeling from Pop's body is still vivid in my hand and my mind.

He loved his jeans. He'd quit wearing them for awhile, saying he was too old for them, but after he got even older, he decided he ought to be able to wear anything he wanted—and he wanted jeans. When John pulled Pop's suit out of his closet at Mayberry, I protested, but he reminded me that his dad liked to look sharp when he stepped out. Reluctantly I agreed, but I still think Pop would have preferred his jeans for eternity.

We found napkins and Kleenex in most of the jacket pockets. Pop always kept them handy to wipe off or wipe up his dribbles. We left them there.

I *hate* that we didn't think to slip in any Little Debbie brownies.

After approving his appearance, we returned to his place. I was cleaning bathrooms—anticipating after-funeral guests—when Sue, a cousin of some degree to John, arrived with the back of her SUV full of food. Not only is she a wonderfully generous and loving person, but she can also carry a conversation all by herself. She reminds me a little of Mary Ann (John's first cousin) that way.

Mom got groggy listening to Sue talk about people she didn't know; she slipped away to the guest room to take a nap. Sue left an hour or so later. After Mom woke up, we asked her to catch the phone while we went to talk to the lawyer who had drawn up Pop's will. John signed more paperwork there.

The viewing was held Thursday evening. We arrived first, of course. Our casket spray was in place; flowers from John's church, from his coworkers and from mine, had all been delivered. The ones from Mayberry Homes started me crying.

Viewings are odd things, being social events structured around death. You talk, you cry, you laugh, you renew acquaintances, while the guest of honor doesn't participate at all.

A lot of people who'd known Pop had already passed away, but about forty people were still around to pay their respects. Mark was so shaky he needed to use his cane. His wife, Lillian, was with him, as were Mark, Jr., his wife and their three kids.

Kellie surprised us and drove down from Garland with a card signed by all of the ladies. She said everyone at House 2 would gather on the porch Friday morning, and when the funeral service started at 10:30, they would fling birdseed in honor of Pop. Made me cry—no surprise.

Brother S is a popular minister in the Whitehouse area. Frankly, John and I don't care for him, but that's neither here nor there. Pop liked him; Pop wanted him; Pop got him. Brother S asked the guests for information and stories so he could prepare the eulogy. Someone immediately mentioned the big rubber snake Pop used to scare people with—he always did like a practical joke. Several other people offered stories, too.

After the viewing, Kellie followed us back to the house, curious to see where he had grown up and had lived most of his life. John described the property as it used to be and filled in a lot of images for her. We gave her two of Pop's small concrete birds to place in the garden in front of House 2.

Later that night, when Charlie exhibited pre-seizure behavior, I gave him some extra medicine, then slept on the floor with him pressed up next to me. I hadn't been sleeping well, so floor or bed didn't make much difference to me.

We were up early Friday morning for our walk. It was wonderfully cool—real actual autumn cool—but just half an hour later, the humidity increased and the temperature started climbing.

Since Charlie's used to being by himself at Mom's apartment, we decided it'd be easier for him to stay there, rather than having him upset by so many strange people moving around Pop's house after the funeral.

He seemed to breathe a sigh of relief when we got to her place—he knew what that was about. I took him for another short walk; when he knew we were leaving, he retreated to her bedroom and settled down. He probably slept the entire time we were gone.

Mom decided not to go to the cemetery. She said someone needed to let in the ladies from Pleasant Hill Baptist Church after the service. They had already delivered a truckload of food.

John and I left for the cemetery. It's only about three miles from the house, but it seemed to take forever to get there. It's at the end of a long, winding, rough, potholed road…an analogy to life if you think about it.

To the left of the cemetery gate, a short way in, and under old shade trees are the graves of Pop's mother and father. To the left of their graves is Mother Pat's grave. The double-wide headstone she and Pop now share was already engraved with his name and birth date. It only awaited his date of death.

To the left of the graves, the funeral home had erected a royal blue canopy, and set up several rows of folding chairs with plush, royal-blue chair covers. The silver of the casket reflected the blues, making them shimmer, so the casket looked like a boat sailing in a sea of its own reflection.

People began arriving. Susan, Springcreek's associate pastor, made the long drive from Garland out of respect for John and to represent the church. After everyone was seated, John and I were still looking for his cousin Mary Ann. She hadn't come to the viewing; can't remember why. The service had just barely started when she and her husband and mother hurried into the cemetery and sat in the back row.

The service began with a recording of "Amazing Grace." As the tape played, I sat with head bowed, trying to fight back the tears rolling down my cheeks, losing the battle, but hoping no one would notice—I hate crying in front of people—because at least I wasn't making much noise except for snuffling.

John had put plenty of Kleenex in his jacket pockets—but he'd taken his jacket off and left it in the car before the service started because it was just too hot to wear. I had only two tissues on me. The first one was already completely soggy; the other was way past its prime.

Then Brother S started speaking. That dried up my tears fast. His eulogy sounded jerky and pathetic, like he was reading his notes from the night before. He said Pop was survived by a son, a brother, and grandkids—Pop doesn't have any grandkids. At least he mentioned the birdseed-flinging ceremony taking place at Mayberry, which made me smile.

Eulogy over. People mingled, but I remember very little of it. While John was talking with someone, I spotted Mary Ann. I had been mostly OK up till then, but as I approached her and said her name, my voice broke…and I just crumpled.

Mary Ann is tiny; probably half my height and a third my weight. We aren't close, yet there I was, clinging to her, sobbing into her shoulder. I don't know why her nearness broke me.

I finally managed to pull back— shielding my nose from view. It was getting messy. "I hope you have some Kleenex in your purse." She did, thank goodness.

Mary Ann and I joined John and funeral-man Steve at the casket. Since she hadn't been able to come to the viewing, we had arranged for the lid to be raised to allow her to say good-bye to Pop. I stepped around to one end and from that angle, looking at the top of his head, it did seem like he was sleeping. His last haircut, which I had given him, had just started growing out.

John and I were last to leave, finally allowing the waiting undertakers to do the rest of their job. Almost everyone from the cemetery had gathered at the house, where the church ladies were already getting food on the table. They suggested I go in the living room and relax, so I did. I pulled up a little foot stool and sat next to Mom.

People ate (except for Mark); people talked; people laughed; people went home. When we were alone again, I quickly cleaned up the kitchen, then Mom and I headed over to her place to get Charlie, stopping first at the cemetery. The grave had been filled in and covered with flowers.

I hadn't seen it when we arrived, but going back through the cemetery gate, I glanced down—and saw a bright, shiny, new nickel. It made me think of Pop's habit of checking the coin return slots of every pay phone or newspaper machine he passed. I've heard of pennies from heaven, but nickels?

It made me feel better to think so. "Hey, Pop—"

John and I drove home Saturday morning, ate a quick lunch, and went to Mayberry to finish cleaning out the room. It was sad, but not as difficult as we'd feared.

John gave Kellie his Bible, which pleased her. She had often seen him reading it.

He gave Pop's old pocketknife—he'd carried one all his life—to Michael.

Gabriella asked for his bolo tie and the small glass that held the toothpicks he collected. Pop liked a toothpick after he ate—why I don't know since most of his real teeth were gone.

Cortney picked out one of his belt buckles, engraved with her birth year.

John has his dad's Masonic ring. Pop had it for so long that it's almost worn through in places.

He'd worn a cord and whistle around his neck for the last ten months, to blow for help if he needed it. I have that.

So. How are we doing? Mostly all right, I guess. Because Pop went quickly, he had very little pain. We take comfort in that.

John's faith is strong; he finds peace in that. I suppose I find comfort in John's peace.

But I sure miss that old man.

Sunday, August 19:

Since the funeral...

Charlie hadn't shown any interest in going to Mayberry since Pop died—it's like he knew Grampy wasn't there anymore. However, last week he chose to walk to the shopping-strip parking lot that's kitty-corner from it.

We passed a dog grooming place, complete with faux fire hydrant in a grassy area out front where Charlie likes to "read" the mail. Then we walked by the burger joint where Pop and I had lunch a couple of times. At the pay phone that stands near its entrance, I stuck my finger into the coin return slot in honor of his habit of checking for change. I half-hoped to find a new nickel like the one at the cemetery, but the slot was empty.

Charlie and I walked on a little further—maybe five feet to the end of the sidewalk. And there, right in front of us, was a beat-up, old, worse-for-wear nickel. "Ho Ho, Pop," I thought. "First you send a shiny one at the grave, and now this worn-out one near the old folks home."

Finding that old nickel made me smile through my tears. Listen, John and I both have unpredictable weepy moments, but mostly I find that when I think of Pop, I smile. The sadness is there, but I remember the pleasant times we had together, or the funny things he said or did—and I smile. Sometimes my eyes fill with tears, but still I smile. This was one of those times.

And now a final story.

The cemetery memorial Pop had wanted to attend was held yesterday. John and I decided to drive down Friday and spend the night. We hadn't had any rain for months, but Friday morning, we no sooner pulled away from the curb than it started raining. It down-poured on us almost all the way to Tyler. At times it got so dark it was like night had fallen—only worse because the headlights didn't illuminate anything but rain.

It rained the rest of the day and into the night, finally stopping early Saturday morning—but then starting again just before it was time to go to the cemetery for the memorial service.

The thunder freaked out Charlie; we decided I would stay with him, and John would go to the service alone.

By the time he returned to the house, the storm had stopped. We took advantage of the dry spell to get the Olds packed up. We were almost out of town before it started raining once again. It rained almost all the way back to Garland, but we needed it, and we were glad to be going home.

I think Pop, too, was glad to go "Home" at last…leaving his old, beaten-up, worse-for-wear nickel body to live in his bright, shiny and new one.

A FEW MORE COMMENTS FROM RUBBERSTAMPERS

Barb: Please keep us posted on Pop's condition. I feel as if he's my Grandpa from all of the stories that you've shared.
Libby
***

Re: Pop is gone

I miss him too, Flossie. I never met Pop in person, but I felt I knew him by your posts of his trials, triumphs, humor and human-ness. Pop for me lived through your eyes and your loving words—and still does.
Ellen
***

I never pass a Little Debbie snack display without thinking of Pop.
Linda
***

Thank you for opening up and sharing this wonderful man with us. It came at the perfect time for me, and I now know that I can do what I have to in the coming months.
Jann
***

So many things of his last few days reminded me of my husband's last days—the arched eyebrows, the toothless smile, the picking at the sheets. Until you shared Pop, I didn't understand what was happening, and had no one to ask. In your grief, you have given me a precious gift: a peace and comfort I have not known before. Thank you.
Sandy
***

Your letters about Pop have touched my soul so much. Like many others I feel he belongs to all of us. Saying goodbye to my own daddy will be hard, but your letters of Pop have helped prepare me for that time to come.
Cindy
***

Postscript: All of Pop's Mayberry ladies have passed on now, as have Mark, Mary Ann, Charlie, my dad, and my sister. Miss Margaret recovered from her colon cancer, and she and Dianne are still going strong. As is my mom.

www.ingramcontent.com/pod-product-compliance
Lightning Source LLC
Chambersburg PA
CBHW020915290526
45784CB00002BA/557